Wa... A Fine Line

Darren,
All the best in your future
adventures as you press on)!

Kathy

Order this book online at www.trafford.com/08-1165
or email orders@trafford.com

Most Trafford titles are also available at major online book retailers.

Note for Librarians: A cataloguing record for this book is available from Library
and Archives Canada at www.collectionscanada.ca/amicus/index-e.html

Printed in Victoria, BC, Canada.

ISBN: 978-1-4251-8665-4

*We at Trafford believe that it is the responsibility of us all, as both individuals
and corporations, to make choices that are environmentally and socially sound.
You, in turn, are supporting this responsible conduct each time you purchase a
Trafford book, or make use of our publishing services. To find out how you are
helping, please visit www.trafford.com/responsiblepublishing.html*

*Our mission is to efficiently provide the world's finest, most comprehensive
book publishing service, enabling every author to experience success.
To find out how to publish your book, your way, and have it available
worldwide, visit us online at www.trafford.com/10510*

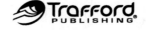

www.trafford.com

North America & international
toll-free: 1 888 232 4444 (USA & Canada)
phone: 250 383 6864 ◆ fax: 250 383 6804
email: info@trafford.com

The United Kingdom & Europe
phone: +44 (0)1865 487 395 ◆ local rate: 0845 230 9601
facsimile: +44 (0)1865 481 507 ◆ email: info.uk@trafford.com

10 9 8 7 6 5 4 3 2

WALKING A FINE LINE

Pressing On
Through Chronic Illness:
~ A Memoir ~

Kathy McWhirter

~For teachers past, present and future~

Acknowledgements

Writing this book has been both exhilarating and terrifying; but I could not have done it without the support of family, friends, and caring people who took this project seriously. You are my lifeline to the world, and I offer you my sincere thanks for clarifying events, providing pertinent information, and filling in the gaps.

My beautiful daughters, Rachel and Becky, have given inspiration and a listening ear to my ramblings. My brother Mike patiently read the first unedited chapters and helped immensely. Without fanfare, my close friend Bernadette gave me the words I needed to hear. "Just do it, Kathy. Start writing." So the journey began.

Thank-you to my best friend of thirty-three years, Kelly-Leigh, for believing in me in so many ways. Thanks to Kristin, for helping me grow in my faith, and to Helene, my pen pal and great encourager. Thanks to Alison, creative super mom that you are, for being there for me. Thank-you to all the teachers that have touched my life, nurturing and building up an injured soul into a strong, confident human being.

Upon completing the first draft, I had no idea how much more work was ahead, but with key people to guide me, my sanity remained intact! Thank-you Jo, Barb, Jim, Kelly-Leigh, Velma and Sally Jennings for your suggestions and help with editing. Velma, you're a star! I am indebted to all who responded to my queries, providing articles, pictures and answers for my research. Thank-you to the amazing people at the Multiple Sclerosis Society of Canada, especially for the literature you provide to people like me, who need it the most.

~ THE HARDEST PART ~

Everyday I walk a fine line
So sure I can beat the odds, it's Gods
Will, not mine to decide
The hardest part is feeling so fine
And then crossing over the fine line
Invisible to visible
Denial to recognition

My body knows the secret
And betrays my thoughts; it's not
As bad as you might think
The hardest part is feeling so weak
The tremors in my legs catch up with me
Frustration to patience
Stranger to friend

My spirit has an answer
Acceptance helps the pain; it's gain
In moving towards peace
The hardest part is identity
Crossing over, crossing back is confusion
for me
Disbelief to belief
Despair to hope

Preamble

This book has been the culmination of many things. First, it was born out of a desire to write. The idea of a story about living with chronic illness grew into so much more. Secondly, as timing is critical, so it was with this writing – it was the right time. Thirdly, I had friends who encouraged me and believed I could do it. It was fuel for the fire.

The story begins in 1994, after the birth of my second daughter, and at times delves further into the past. My tendency to ramble and say it all in one breath was challenged repeatedly. I have learned lessons about clarity and conciseness. Just as I get out of bed each morning, slowly, stiffly and tentatively, the writing began...

Multiple Sclerosis has been an unwelcome visitor in my life for ten years, changing everything for better and worse. The better is that I am doing something I love (writing), and I am living in Victoria BC, a place that is hospitable to the elderly, sick and lame. The worse is that I can hike up mountains and ski down them only in my dreams, and that some days I feel like I'm living in the body of a ninety-year old. Unfortunately, that is often the nature of disease. I strive to rise above.

The chronic-illness community has a small but powerful voice and my hope is that in these pages you will find the inspiration to carry on, no matter what your disability. We all have a story to tell. We can make a difference.

Blessings!

Kathy McWhirter
September 2008

ONE

"You are a child of the universe,
no less than the trees and the stars,
you have a right to be here."
~ Desiderata ~

The doctor raised her voice above the wail of a newborn baby. "It's a girl," she said with a smile in her voice. I was ecstatic, filled with a sense of triumph on the birth of our second daughter, almost eight years after the first. The crowning glory was a natural labour that came unexpectedly after having a Caesarean for the first delivery. I wanted to dance down the hallways and tell the whole world. The odds of natural childbirth were not good but I had beaten them and now had a gorgeous healthy child.

Months later, as I lifted one leaden foot in front of the other to reach the crying baby upstairs, I thought about the joy that had quickly turned to exhaustion. By day, our new daughter was a typical infant: sleeping, bottle/breast feeding, creating a mountain of diapers, occasionally crying and mostly growing. By night, she was a discontented creature who woke frequently, cried incessantly and wore me down to the bone. I dreaded nighttime. My jangled nerves worked overtime and screamed in protest as the baby screamed. I had wanted her so badly, but the cost to the family had been more than I had bargained for.

The long cold days of winter were taking their toll. One night after numerous trips to the crib, I felt desperate. Walking downstairs with my crying baby, I glanced out of the backdoor window at the piles of soft white snow, glistening and beckoning to me. How easy it would be, I thought, to open the door and lie down in the snow, so peaceful and quiet. Another part of my brain scorned the idea, knowing the baby would scream louder and I would scream too. I shook my head to clear the fog, and carefully went down the stairs, clutching my precious baby. Exhaustion plays tricks on the mind, I counselled myself. Finally, the baby began sleeping through the night but even with adequate sleep, I was still exhausted.

In the spring of 1995, my husband John David (who went by either name, but I married Dave) was keen to start his own campground business in Robb, in the foothills of West Central Alberta. I was sad to give up my seasonal job working for the Provincial Forestry Department, but I had agreed that a new baby and a business would be more than enough work for me.

There was so much to do to get started. By July, we were set up with a fifth-wheel camping trailer to live in that would have been ideal except for the endless rain, a crying baby, and no customers. "Lovett River" was a small government campground, leased to us annually, with rustic facilities and in what most would consider the "back country." Dave made plans to build a group shelter and buy a couple of tipis (teepees) for a "novel camping experience."

Such good ideas fit our lifestyle well, except for my doubts about the location. It was out of the way for most travellers though the people who came appreciated the remote feel of the area. The first summer dragged on and my fatigue deepened, especially when I knew we were operating the business at a loss even though all our business planning told us this was a typical beginning.

"I'm out of shape after the birth of a baby," I told everyone. "Regular exercise is the key." Since I had always been an active, high-energy person, the idea of pulling myself out of this slump appealed to me. I was motivated. Now I had to find what would work with our busy lifestyle and a baby. I decided I would walk and push the stroller.

The weather had improved so I marched up the street; my neighbour watched curiously. Beautiful surroundings distracted me from my nagging thoughts as a rutted pathway led from our street to a paved highway. Looking westward, an expanse of forested hills quickly turned into large angular rocks that jutted into the sky forming the spectacular backdrop of the Rocky Mountains. The highway dipped into a valley, climbed a hill around the bend, and then disappeared into rich, dark green coniferous trees, with contrasting lighter hues of alder and poplar.

I recalled idyllic early morning bicycle trips of only a few years ago on that highway. Those were special times where I connected my physical and spiritual self to the power of Mother Nature. I breathed in clean cool air, listened to birds singing and water rippling in the nearby Embarrass River. White-tailed and mule deer often crossed my path; beautiful, graceful creatures that bolted into the trees at the first rumble of traffic. Pavement ended when the highway turned south into the Forestry Trunk Road, where dust and gravel made riding unpleasant. I turned around at this point and retraced my route. Northward, the highway went sixty kilometres to Edson, with a population of five thousand. There were approximately two hundred people in Robb.

We lived in an area known as the Coal Branch, where coal mining had been a way of life since the early 1900s.

The area included small towns such as Edson, Robb, Mercoal, and Cadomin, which still exist. Communities had come and gone over the years, such as Coalspur, Lovettville and Mountain Park. Currently, three coalmines operate in a hundred-kilometre radius, found on the "Branch." I had heard it described many times as "God's country," and although it was isolated, its spectacular rugged beauty was a trademark and sought after by many nature lovers, hunters, anglers and campers. Pioneers of our country grew up here, tough, spirited men and women who cherished the land.

"Car!" my little daughter Becky shouted, bringing me back to the present. We walked east along the highway toward the access road that led into the hamlet of Robb. I glanced north into the ditch at the power line right-of-way that led to paths made by man and animal. We had cross-country skied in this area during the snowy winter months and discovered where underground coal burned, so I steered clear of the soft, potentially dangerous site. I pushed the stroller off the pavement as a large truck passed. The horn blared. I looked up and waved at the driver, who tipped his hat and grinned from ear to ear.

"Look, Becky, at the pretty flowers." The noisy truck was in the distance. A couple of bright orange tiger lilies danced in the breeze, a local wild flower picked too often. We turned towards the tiny town and took the shortest route home. I was tired. I knew it would be worth it, though. In a couple of weeks, my stamina and strength would increase and the payoff would be a sense of well-being and less fatigue.

The fall season brought a welcome change of routine for all of us. The campground drew a few hardy types in the cooler weather, as well as hunters, who usually preferred to be further in the bush and on their own.

Dave managed the business while I took care of family and bookkeeping.

Our oldest daughter, Rachel, attended one of the last two-room schoolhouses in the province at the start of grade three. Her teacher and I had become friends. Bernadette was finishing a maternity leave after the birth of her first child and we had a chance to get to know one another during this time. I recalled the hike we went on together in the spring after Ben was born. Becky was still small and light and I carried her on my back in an aluminum-frame baby carrier that gave her a bird's-eye view over my shoulder.

"It's a perfect day for a walk. The air smells so good." My friend had a few hours of freedom from the needs of her newborn son.

"It's an amazing place," Bernadette replied as she looked at the forest and rolling hills, and drank in the cool, clean air. We told stories and laughed as we trudged along. I kept hoisting the pack around. How could one little baby feel so heavy?

"Are you okay, Kathy?"

"I think so; I'm just so out of shape." We stopped for a rest but it was a huge effort to finish the journey. More than ten years have passed since then, and I still remember the beauty of the day and a friendship marred by inexplicable exhaustion.

Our home was heated with a wood-burning stove, so Dave and I had the daunting task of cutting and hauling enough firewood to last the winter. After a cool, wet summer, the fall had turned warm and dry. We brought Becky with us, which made the slow laborious work even slower.

Our method was to scout the site for the perfect tree, usually pine or spruce. Cut the tree down. Cut off the branches and pull them out of the way. Wear work

17

gloves. Buck the tree into lengths of less than eighteen inches. Carry the wood to the truck. Stack the wood carefully in order to haul the maximum amount home. Stop for a smoke break (not me, thank goodness I quit) and file the chainsaw. Start all over with the next tree. Get sticky sap stuck on your hands and clothes, and wood bits down your shirt. The smell of freshly cut wood was mixed with gasoline fumes. I dashed between the truck and Becky, loading what wood I was able. When we got home, it had to be carefully stacked and covered with a tarp. Sometimes Rachel helped.

"Aww, Mom, do I have to? It's so heavy," she protested as I began making dinner.

"Yes, your father could use the help. Make sure you're wearing old clothes." A huge level stump was used as a chopping block during the winter, and Dave split most of the larger wood with a maul and wedge, which my 120-pound frame did not have the power or muscle to do, but I enjoyed splitting wood with an axe. There was plenty to split each winter.

"I'm off to the meeting!" I yelled as I ran out the door in a rush to make the Sunday evening fire department meeting. Joining as a volunteer fire fighter was one of the best decisions I had made when we moved to Robb, even though I had only a faint idea of the commitment involved. It caused conflict in my marriage and stress at the worst times. However, I loved the action and learning how tools and equipment worked, as well as the satisfaction of helping people in the community.

"Tonight we'll work on rescue carries and drags," the training officer said. "First there's a video before we practise some of the moves." A couple of firefighters backed the fire trucks out of the building to make more room, and the video started. It was a review for most of us, but with only a dozen or so emergency calls a year, hands-on training kept us current. There were few structural fires. The majority of the calls involved vehicles, and as first responders to the scene, our department was trained in vehicle extrication and first aid.

The crew was mostly men. This was familiar to me because my father and two brothers had been my recreational companions in my youth and tools, equipment and vehicles were standard fare. It was interesting to learn how these things worked. I was soon to see just how well our new "jaws of life" worked in a context I never dreamed possible.

~~~~~~

Winter had taken hold one cold December morning when I set out to Edson to run errands and pick up supplies. It was about minus fifteen degrees Celsius, and the surrounding countryside was frozen and snow covered. Most of the time the main roads were ploughed, but this did not always make them less slippery. Usually, the cold provided more traction. It was a full daytrip to two towns, and I left my baby daughter, Becky, at home with Dave. She usually came with me.

We had purchased a small station wagon months before. It was front-wheel drive - smooth and powerful - but it did not prevent my dislike of winter driving. I slowed down at a few slippery sections, but highway traffic was light and shift change from the coalmine workers, who used the road daily, had already passed through.

Brrrr, I shivered. It was cold. Grey low-lying clouds added to the winter gloom. I went to the accountant's office, signed the necessary papers and finished other errands quickly. The highway to Hinton was bare and dry, and after a lunch break, I began the many trips in and out of stores and offices. Christmas lights brightened the dullness and I forced a cheeriness I did not feel. As usual, I was exhausted but it felt good to finish most of the items on the list. I headed for home with the car packed with groceries, gifts and the empty baby car seat. I came home via a gravel logging road, used and maintained by the local pulp mill and open to the public year round. Sharing a road with huge loaded logging trucks was unnerving, but with business taken care of in Edson and then Hinton, it was the fastest, most practical route home.

At about 4 pm, the light was fading to a sort of "flat light," the kind that made it difficult to pick out fine detail. I had never liked skiing in those conditions, either. A sea of white and grey enveloped me and I squinted in concentration.

"Almost home," I thought with relief as I rounded the icy corner. Then ahead I saw a loaded logging truck coming towards me. It surprised me, because I had not encountered any trucks earlier. I do not remember if I pressed hard on the brakes, but I probably did. I was suddenly in a skid headed straight towards the truck, out of control. The car seemed to speed up and I kept my eyes wide open as I slammed into the front driver's side of the massive truck, spun around in a wild 180-degree turn, and landed in the ditch on the opposite side of the road. The logging truck driver had seen I was having trouble controlling the vehicle. He slowed down to a crawl and pulled over as much as he dared. The loaded truck dumped onto its side, and spilled logs into the ditch opposite me. The driver, unhurt, scrambled out of the cab. He came to find me, certain I was dead.

All I could think about was how this had happened. I waited. Where was the fire department, of which I was a member, with their equipment and rescue tools? I was pinned against the steering wheel and the console looked like an accordion. Shock set in as someone covered me with a blanket and cold numbed my senses as my body registered the trauma, and I shook violently. The rest was a blur. The fire department, bystanders, my husband, ambulance and police all came to do their part. I was put on a spinal board after being pulled from the mangled car. It felt like steel - cold, hard and impersonal. The Jaws of Life was not needed after all because the driver's door was only jammed in tight and took a bit of force to open. There was no blood, only a sharp pain in my lower left side.

"Ma'am, we need to ask you a few questions," said the ambulance attendant as we headed for the hospital. "What speed were you going when this happened? Was there anyone travelling with you? What have you eaten today? Did you consume any alcoholic beverages before you drove home?" The questions droned on. Once again, I was asked if I had been drinking. There was an invisible knife in my ribs and my back was numb.

"We're sorry, but we have to ask you this," said the person in the uniform. I got mad.

"I told you already, I was not drinking!" Thank goodness that was true, because we used to do it all the time in our younger days and with my family's history of alcoholism weighing heavily on me, I was careful about my actions and behaviour toward alcohol. "Moderation in all things, including moderation," my dad often said. I was so grateful my daughters were at home safe with Dave.

The accident was my fault. It took me weeks to come to terms with that fact, but I hit the logging truck, not the other way around. The actions of the logging truck driver possibly saved my life. Perhaps I was driving too fast for the conditions. I will never know. It was out of my control. At the time, it was extremely icy in the area, which people at the scene attested to. I am thankful to be alive to tell the story and to have suffered only a couple of broken ribs and a collapsed lung.

The car was destroyed and sat in our driveway to haunt me for a long time before it was finally towed away. The baby car seat that was directly behind me on the backseat was crushed and bent (the way I walked for many weeks after) and was a constant reminder of how miraculous it was that I was still alive, and that my daughter had been placed out of harm's way.

Dave was very upset with me. Even though he helped me recognize the accident was my fault, it was not done kindly. Technically, the baby car seat should have been placed in the middle of the backseat, not where I had it strapped directly behind me, and if Becky had been with me on that fateful day, she would probably have been killed. Dave never let me forget. He was angry with me for wrecking one of the nicest cars we had ever owned, even though it was properly insured and money eventually came our way to replace it. Dave pointed out the actions of the logging truck driver saved my life, and I agreed with him and wrote to the driver to thank him. Our already strained marriage was as taut as wire from years of misunderstanding.

Christmas was bittersweet. I felt surrounded by the love of concerned family and friends and yet there was an undercurrent of tension in our house. The slow start to the campground business we had undertaken the previous summer was discouraging. Dave was consumed by planning and operating the home-based business and I was on the sidelines, willing to help but not willing to put the business first. I tried, but to me a job was part of life, not everything in life. I really missed the friendship, income and independence that my seasonal Forestry job had provided – it gave me a sense of pride, rather than fear that I had done something wrong.

Under the Christmas tree was a book for Dave from our good friends, David and Helene, who had moved across the country the previous year to Nova Scotia. The author's name caught my attention, "Norman Vincent Peale" and I recalled seeing that name on a book lying around our house when I was growing up. The book was "The Power of Positive Thinking," and my Dad often referred to the wisdom found there.

The new book was entitled, "A Treasury of Courage and Confidence," and being intrigued, I began to read. Dave did not seem interested. The theme was believing in yourself, trusting in God, and learning how to cope with life's obstacles and challenges. The timing could not have been better. I was still recovering from the car accident and trying hard to come to terms with all that had happened, while fighting the insidious "poor me" voice inside.

The book was filled with indisputable wisdom, short stories, verses and quotes from famous and ordinary people, Scripture, and Peale's rock-solid philosophy on positive creative living. When I read that sometimes God has to allow circumstances to put us on our back, literally, so that we may be forced to look up and regard Him and what His plan is for us, I felt immediate recognition. Returning to the passage, I became sure that God must exist and that it was not just a freak series of coincidences that kept me alive. I lost track of the fact that it was not my book, marking passages and reading, reading, reading.

One day after Christmas, the phone rang.

"Hi ya, Kath, how are you feeling? Would February be too soon for a visit?" my father asked.

23

"Wow, that would be great. I'm feeling a lot better now that I've stopped walking hunched over," I laughed. "It won't be too cold for you?" Dad suffered from undetermined heart problems.

"Oh no, I'll just bring some warmer clothes," he said casually.

"I'll pick you up at the airport, if you'll let me know the dates." It was a three-hour drive to the airport, and I suspected my "close call" had something to do with the visit, but I welcomed the chance to spend time together because our visits had been infrequent and random over my adult life. I loved his wisdom, outlook, and humour. The week flew by and Dad's energy and appetite surprised me, but not his usual good spirits. I cherished our time together.

My own physical and mental health was much improved and I felt fully recovered from the accident by April. Therefore, when I found out the Robb Ranger Station was slated to close permanently at the end of the year, my resolve to be a "stay at home" mom weakened. It would be my last chance to work locally for the Alberta Forest Service for the summer of 1996. With ten years of prior service in a variety of seasonal jobs in Robb, Hinton and Edson, many of the friends and contacts I had made would be lost after the closure.

Our small business operating a campground had been very slow the summer before, and I knew Dave could handle it himself if I were needed elsewhere. I carefully brought the subject up, expecting a big argument.

At first, he was adamant.

"We agreed, Kathy, if you were to have another baby you would stay at home and help with the business," Dave stated.

"I know, but I didn't know the Robb Ranger Station would be closing its doors in this community forever!

24

Plus, we could really use the money." It was a strong argument. We rallied back and forth for several days, and finally Dave suggested I propose to work part-time - maybe thirty hours a week instead of forty. I was sceptical at first, although this idea had benefits to both employer and employee. Forestry would save money. I would make money but not be burdened with a full-time job.

It worked! At first, my boss was opposed to the idea of changing my work hours from the standard forty that I had worked in previous summers, but I think it fit into his tight budget for the season. I convinced him I could still perform all my duties in less time.

The funny job title was "Forest Guardian" which most people assumed to be "Ranger" as soon as they saw the forestry uniform and truck. It had elements of a ranger's job, but was specific to the operation and maintenance of four to six district campgrounds. It was a "jack of all trades" job, which I loved. I wore the same uniform as the Area Forest Rangers and drove a green Alberta Forest Service truck from site to site in a 60-kilometre radius, collecting camping fees, providing information to the public and performing general maintenance. I was issued bright orange coveralls and a pair of work gloves, along with some basic tools and a toilet scrub brush. Even though each area had janitorial and maintenance staff, we were expected to perform the "grunt" work when and where necessary. It took a certain amount of self-motivation and a love of the outdoors, people and hard work.

A controversial part of the job was enforcement. I became frustrated with how little power we guardians had to enforce the regulations set out by the Alberta Forest Service and contained in the Forestry Act. We carried copies of these in our truck and had to follow them. This sometimes caused problems.

Most of the rules were basic common sense. Thou shalt not steal, vandalize, burn down the forest, ride off-highway-vehicles in the campground, or have loud wild parties at two in the morning. Telling someone who has already decided to break the rules to stop doing so is not much of a threat. My options were limited. In an emergency, the ranger on call or police could drive out to the site but this would usually take an hour, given the back road locations. Usually I took names and/or licence plate numbers to report. The system was inadequate and ineffective. Normally the problems were minor, but when I found out the seasonal guardians were required to obtain "special constable" status for the 1996 season, I was thrilled. Six years of compromising was about to change!

The weeklong training took place in Hinton at the Forest Technology School and renewed my enthusiasm. As I prepared my truck for the season in early May, I thought I would finally be able to do my job effectively. I would make a difference, kick butt, and be taken seriously.

Preparing for the season, I put the tailgate down and climbed into the back of the truck. Shocked at how stiff my legs and back felt, I looked around furtively and hoped I was alone. The stiffness never went away no matter how hard I worked or how much firewood I hauled. I blamed it on impending middle age even though forty was two years away. In the back of my mind, I suspected there was something wrong.

A thunderstorm swept in unexpectedly, bringing torrents of rain and making a sloppy mess of the roads. Huge potholes turned into pools of liquid mud and I gritted my teeth as the road changed from soft and slippery to bone jarring. I saw a flash of lightening in the distant black sky and automatically started counting: one-one thousand, two-one thousand, three-one thousand... At ten, there was a rumble of thunder and I knew lightening was about ten kilometres away. Rain turned to a trickle and the storm moved westward. As I drove into Fairfax Lake campground I heard a loud "kwuk, kwuk" followed by a long falsetto wail. Another cry pierced the air as a pair of loons skimmed the surface of the still water and landed in a flurry.

A single truck camper was parked in a stall on the first tier adjacent to the lake. I checked the beach/dock area, bathrooms, and pay station before heading up the hill to the Forestry cabin. I was looking forward to an early night and a good sleep.

The following morning dawned crisp and clear and I took my time preparing for the day. My shift started at 1.30 pm. After a leisurely breakfast and quiet reading time, I decided to walk out to the unpaved, bumpy highway on the gravel access road. I was surprised how dry it was, except for one section at the bottom of the hill. Tiny, wild strawberry plants hugged the gravelly soil beside the road, and I stopped to look for the flavourful, sweet berries but there were none. Blueberries were much more prolific that year, so I scanned for the twiggy low-lying shrubs, dreaming about the delicious pies these berries made. They were tiny and took a long time to pick. I learned huckleberries were a local favourite, bigger and juicer than wild blueberries, and I looked for patches of these instead after a friend had pointed out the bushes.

As I walked back to the cabin, my pace slowed and my legs became heavy. By the end of the walk, I could barely lift my feet – it was as if a brick was tied to each foot. Why couldn't I get myself in shape?

The rest of the summer continued in the same fashion.

I started out feeling fine but then tiredness would storm in and I was forced to stop and rest. I began driving my truck up and down the hill to the lake, campsites, washrooms and firewood bins instead of walking. We were busy that summer and with a full schedule, I adapted to the lack of energy however I could, not really noticing the effect as I adjusted to the changes in my body.

September was glorious. The campgrounds were quiet again. I painted picnic tables, cleaned firewood bins and installed new hardware in bathrooms. The fish-cleaning stand by the dock reeked of fish guts and flies buzzed overhead as I quickly bagged the offending parts, and placed the double bags carefully in the back of the truck. As I raked woodchips and stacked wood I was suddenly very tired, so I finished slowly before heading for home.

I was just starting dinner when the phone rang.

"Kathy, it's Auntie Jean," the voice said. My aunt lived in Toronto and we rarely spoke on the phone, so it was strange that she was calling.

"Are you sitting down, dear? I've got some bad news." I tensed, not at all prepared for what I was about to hear.

"Your mother was found dead in the house today. I'm so sorry." My mind went blank. I could not speak.

"Kathy, are you there?" she asked as I attempted to answer.

"What hap-p-pened?" Auntie Jean was very matter-of-fact. She told me mom had been drinking heavily since the death of her second husband nine months earlier, and her heart had given out. Why was I so shocked? Mom's drinking had destroyed many things in her life and friends had predicted this result.

I put down the phone and began to sob, wishing I had paid closer attention to my mother's frantic phone calls.

TWO

"Thus it is that my friends have made
the story of my life."
~ Helen Keller ~

I had never lost anyone close to me. It was strange and did not seem real at first. I was in a panic to get to Toronto, even though my relatives and people in charge assured me "there is no rush."

Dave and I decided the best way to handle the situation was for me to fly to Toronto on my own, as most of my mother's family was in Ontario. My brothers lived in Vancouver and flew to meet me there. Dave had planned a trip to Vancouver at this time for a high school reunion and offered to take Becky with him. We arranged for Rachel to stay with friends in Robb and continue going to school.

I was on autopilot. The next few days were a blur of emotion, activity and exhaustion. Once I got to Toronto, I slept in the big old house where my mom had died, which everybody thought was weird. Where else was I going to stay? I was familiar with the neighbourhood, most of the arrangements were being made locally, and I refused to incur more cost than necessary by staying in a big, impersonal hotel. There were so many details to be taken care of and it really made sense to be close by.

My mother died in her bedroom while on a drinking binge, with the television blaring and Chinese food in the oven. There she remained for five days. The stark reality of what she had become hit me hard and I kept thinking about how lonely and scared she must have been. Caught in a vicious cycle with nowhere to escape except the bottle, she must have been desperate. I tried to banish the guilt.

"God grant me the serenity to accept the things I cannot change, the courage to change the things I can, and the wisdom to know the difference." Serenity, courage, and wisdom – these were elusive qualities in a suffering alcoholic. The A.A. prayer my mother had sent me eight years before was buried in an old box in the basement. Her dry years did not last. Wisdom and resolve were lost deep in the bottle and Mom was powerless to change her destructive pattern. Once again, my brothers and I were there to pick up the pieces. She had left us many years ago in Vancouver and now she had left us permanently. For me, the bitterness was replaced by sadness.

On the second morning, I woke up to sunshine. I had finally had the first good sleep since I had heard the news several days before. I was starving. I walked a short distance to the shops to buy a few groceries and get a cup of coffee. My attention was caught by the brilliant shades of orange and red leaves on the lovely old trees in the neighbourhood adjacent to the Humber River. On the return trip, the familiar heaviness in my legs caused me to slow my pace. I attributed my exhaustion to the stress of my mother's death.

The day of the funeral arrived and we did not expect many people.

"Hey Kath, you don't wear high heels much, do you?" my brother joked as we ran about preparing the funeral chapel for guests, as I stumbled several times.

"They're actually a bit big," I replied, making excuses.

I was so tired. I could not wait for this to be over.

We were surprised at the number of people at the service, including my ninety-five year old grandmother, who had enriched my life with nurturing, humour and a sharp wit. My mother was her youngest child. Even though Nana had full care in a nursing home and was losing her memory, her comments led me to believe she knew exactly what was going on. She was very sweet and very funny.

"Do you like my outfit, dear?" she asked with a laugh as she opened her long coat and flashed a beautiful flowered dress. It brought tears to my eyes, as everything did at that time.

~~~~~~

My seasonal job ended when I returned from Toronto, weary and saddened. As time passed, my tears lessened and I realized there was little I could have done to prevent my mother's downward spiral. In some ways, it was a time of healing for my brothers and me because we were forced to confront the past and its effect on us. We had been through a lot, growing up with an alcoholic mother. We found closure in writing our individual stories down on paper and sharing them with each other. My father did not attend the funeral. He had been badly hurt by my mother and he preferred to leave the past behind.

"You couldn't have stopped it, Kathy," my friend said emphatically as we walked along the dusty road back home. "I told you about the Al-Anon program that helps families and friends of alcoholics, and I really think some of the people there could help you."

We had talked about this before, when my mother's alcoholic behaviour had surfaced after a dry period. I knew after everything that had happened I had to accept I could not deal with this on my own. I was stubborn, independent and self-sufficient. I valued these qualities, but now they were working against me. The commitment involved evening trips to town, and I was not keen to drive on the highway in the dark in the winter and I knew Dave would not like it. The trip was 120 kilometres. Many families accepted this as part of the lifestyle and travelled back and forth several times a week, but not us. It was wasteful, costly and unnecessary, according to Dave. I tried very hard not to feel isolated.

My battle with getting in shape and keeping a regular fitness program had long been abandoned. The car accident, working for Forestry, the home-based business and my mother's death had interfered with any sustained activity although there was always plenty to do. My friend Shirley and I decided to walk around town one evening in the fall, for a break from routine.

The community was divided into two parts, the hill and the valley. There were about 200 residents, several dozen houses, a fire hall, general store, hotel, school, curling rink, community hall and lots of trees and bush. Within a couple of blocks we were on the perimeter of town and headed up a gravel road towards the Forestry compound. On the north side, adjacent to the railway, was an abandoned Canadian National Railway camp that had shut down only a year before, when the permanent residents had moved away.

To the south, trees and shrubs hid the Forestry wood yard. I thought with satisfaction of the countless truckloads of firewood I had hauled out of the lot and delivered to various campgrounds over the years. The job required energy, attention and motivation. In pouring rain, the woodpiles were slippery and bark came off in chunks, leaving the logs gleaming and grip-less. The heavy pieces were impossible to lift and I passed over them in favour of lighter wood. Hot weather made the job gruelling and sweaty, as did horseflies, mosquitoes and uninvited wildlife. It was a decent workout no matter what.

"Should we continue to the dump, Kathy, or would you like to turn around here?" Shirley asked. I eyed the boarded-up ranger station and the house sitting beside it.

"Let's head back. It's strange to see empty buildings with boards over the windows. Everything in the warehouse and office will be shipped to Edson. I still can't believe it's been closed down for good."

Five houses surrounded the Ranger Station in a beautiful, private setting and the far house remained occupied as the chief ranger commuted to Edson each day to Forestry Headquarters. The other full-time permanent rangers and their families had moved away, which meant fewer children in the community. The school was in jeopardy of closing and the remaining children would be bussed to Edson. Robb was shrinking and I wondered how the community would survive. With one last glance at the empty buildings, I shivered and turned towards home.

I began to notice the all too familiar heaviness in my legs as I struggled to keep up with Shirley. We passed the general store and the streetlights ended. In the dark I lost my footing and stumbled, and Shirley grabbed my arm. I tripped again. As we neared the hotel where the streetlights began, my balance improved. Difficulty navigating in the dark was not in my imagination. In the warmth and light of our house, I soon forgot about my exhaustion and fleeting loss of balance.

Early one evening in November, the phone rang.

"Hi, Kathy. It's a perfect night for flooding the rink. You up for it?" The only ranger left, my boss in the summer and a volunteer firefighter, wanted me to help him flood our community skating rink.

"I guess it's cold enough, John. Sure I'll meet you at the fire hall at seven." It was minus sixteen degrees Celsius, and perfect weather for a job that allowed us to sharpen our skills using the fire trucks and equipment.

"Radio 1, this is tanker truck 45, how do you read?" I spoke into the microphone as John backed the truck slowly out of the fire hall. "Tanker truck 45 leaving the fire hall to flood the skating rink. We'll let you know when we're back."

"That's copied here, thanks," replied a female voice operating the emergency radio.

The tanker shook and lurched forward as John shifted gears on the manual transmission and we headed to the rink to spray the first thousand gallons of water onto the tarmac. To my surprise there was already a layer of ice.

"Scot and I were out the other night, so I'd like to keep this going if we can." John loved to be outdoors with machinery and equipment.

We hooked up a hose line, turned on the pump and started a fine spray of water at the back of the rink. Our bunker gear, the protective clothing firefighters wear, included insulated boots, coveralls, coat, helmet and gloves that kept us warm in the chilly night. It kept the cold out, but also kept the sweat in during emergency calls that involved heat. We emptied the tank and drove to a pond just outside of town where a culvert allowed us access to water to refill the truck, and we made two more runs before the equipment froze up.

"I guess we'll have to call it a night, Kathy. It's coming along, though, pretty soon the kids will be skating," John said with satisfaction.

"How's the commute into Edson going?" I asked curiously, now that the pump was quiet and we could

34

actually hear each other.

"Oh, pretty good. I've heard there's no funding to reopen the Robb Ranger Station, so I'm not sure what we're going to do." John lived with his wife and teenage daughter on the abandoned property but also owned a house in Grande Prairie, and I knew they were thinking about moving. I would be sad to see them go, but there was nothing keeping them in Robb without employment. The government had undertaken many such closures throughout the province and employees relocated to larger centers or found other jobs. John was hardworking, active in the community, a "doer" as opposed to a "dreamer" and always had a good joke to tell. We would miss him.

Rachel had her tenth birthday that winter. We had a chance to go downhill skiing together, which was a big deal for us because it did not happen very often.

"Who is it again, mom? You know, your friend who's meeting us in Jasper?" Rachel asked.

"Kelly-Leigh, her husband and step-son. Remember I told you Kelly-Leigh and I have been close friends since grade six, and we haven't seen each other for almost ten years. She's been busy with her family and veterinary practice in Ontario and I've been busy with you, Becky, Dad and my forestry job."

"How old is her step-son?" Rachel asked.

"I think he's graduated from high school, so almost an adult. Don't worry. You're a good skier and we can keep up to them. Kelly-Leigh and I skied together when we were kids, so I'm excited to meet them and visit." Rachel was happy to be missing a day of school even if it meant getting up early (not something she enjoyed), and she did not like school much, so this was a perfect break.

We had a wonderful day on the slopes together, and it

was so good to reconnect with an old friend. I did not even have to battle tired legs because each rest on the chairlift was enough to keep me going, and I decided I was imagining a problem that was not there. I felt fit, strong, and sure of my abilities.

My father came for another visit, and this time I really noticed his declining health.

"Are you still on a waiting list for open-heart surgery, Dad? I know a couple of years ago, when it was suggested, you couldn't see the point, but now it seems clear it would really help."

"I think I've accepted the inevitable, Kathy. It's just a matter of 'when' and not 'if' any more." He was so thin, pale and weary. I prayed he would last.

Dave built an attractive gazebo-like group shelter at the campground, with a stone fireplace in the center that was wonderful to sit near after a winter trek on cross-country skis. I have a great picture of Dad standing under the domed roof surrounded by lodge pole pine and glistening white snow, looking out of place in his shiny silver jacket, but smiling all the same.

Occasionally customers would book a night or two in a tipi, one of which had a small "airtight" wood-burning stove, but the small 22-site campground was not used much in the winter. Sometimes we had a family outing in the afternoon, and I challenged myself to ski Dave's homemade cross-country ski trail. It was five kilometres of gentle, flat, groomed track with a few tricky spots through tightly woven, young-growth forest. I started out strong and confident but soon began to have light falls that puzzled me, given my cautious and careful style. In the past, I rarely fell. I was not hurt, just surprised and mildly alarmed at my apparent lack of stamina.

Dave had many creative ideas. "I'd like to try

something new this summer, Kathy. What do think about boat rentals that target Fairfax Lake? Customers often ask me if there is somewhere close they could rent a boat."

"I'm not sure, let me think about it." How could we put more money into a business that was still operating at a loss? It would be our third summer. Dave had built a giant shed that acted as a storefront and had a small inventory, basic camping staples, a small cash float, and brochures that described the services. We had already invested in two tipis, a group shelter, and a small store. Everything we did cost so much without the needed revenue coming in to compensate the outflow. We needed more customers. Maybe boats would be a good draw.

"You know, Dave, we could put in a bid to operate Fairfax Lake Campground, which would be a great fit with the boat idea. Since the Alberta Forest Service no longer runs the campgrounds with their own employees and contracts out the seasonal work, we could add Fairfax Lake Campground to our business. It's only fifteen minutes down the Trunk Road, past Lovett River Campground. I could handle Fairfax, which would free you up to operate Lovett River and the boats. It would generate income, that's for sure." And a ton of work, I said to myself. It would also give us some distance from each other while working towards a common goal. Anyone could apply.

We got the bid. The only drawback was that it included two other small campgrounds, but we dove in headfirst and prepared for a busy season. Dave decided to haul the boats from Lovett River to Fairfax Lake on the weekends after purchasing a boat trailer, which made a lot more rentals that way. Each campground had a self-serve kiosk, so we did not have to be there all the time. Most campers were honest and paid their fees accordingly. I was not afraid of hard work but the schedule was intimidating. At least we each had our own set of duties and were not constantly working side by side. My practical, here and now, let's get it done nature clashed with Dave's perfectionist, visionary outlook that questioned everything and trusted nothing. What little intimacy we had was lost in the details of a long-term plan with no room for change or error. There was little forgiveness, a lot of blame and constant worry.

A shadow of gloom hung over me. I could not seem to think clearly or make even the smallest decision. The doctor suggested depression and as I recalled the events of the past year and my never-ending tiredness, I realized this was probably true. That winter I had made trips to town to see a therapist regarding my exhaustion and marital difficulties, and she suggested my lack of energy was a nutritional imbalance, some kind of absorption problem that we pinpointed to yeast intolerance. I should no longer eat bread, pasta, cookies or crackers. I tried it half-heartedly, along with vitamin supplements. I also tried some of her suggestions to improve my marriage. Nothing made any lasting change. Life just kept on coming and at some point the fog lifted.

May 14, 1997. The snow had melted early in spring that year and the forest was bone dry. Paint was peeling and cracking in the bathroom at Lovett River Campground. The bathrooms in Forestry campgrounds were usually containerized vaults set in the ground, with a concrete pad over the top holding the building in place, which provided a level surface and space to work. I appreciated that fact because painting was not my favourite job. I had done too much of it in the house we had built in Robb. "At least the bathroom did not stink,"

I thought, as I finished the last coat and packed up the supplies.

I glanced in the rear-view mirror as I headed down the long, wide hill and watched a thick trail of dust that I created swirl madly behind me. A large flatbed truck with mining equipment came in the opposite direction. I slowed to a crawl as the dust swallowed the road and I was blinded. The cloud settled slowly as I choked in the fine particles. Finally, with pavement in sight I could wind the window down and breathe normally again, except that I could see smoke in the distance.

Dark smoke puffed into the sky. It did not seem to be the dump burning because it rarely put out any smoke and this was billowing up. On our street, I swerved to miss hitting two water packs lying in the road, which I recognized from the fire department. Our house was empty. The fire hall was deserted. I grabbed my gear and found our fire trucks near the community hall. A forest fire was burning near our town but across the highway and sparks had blown over and started a garage roof on fire. The fire department quickly extinguished the blaze and the crew stood by for other possible starts.

I walked across the highway to where a small group of excited residents gasped and pointed to the smoke.

"Water bombers are on their way! You should see all the fall-out from the trees that are on fire and the hotspots on the ground," someone said. I had seen several people wearing water backpacks marching through the bush, spraying any suspicious fire starts.

Suddenly, the screech of a siren pierced the air.

"Get out the way! That was a warning for a water drop near here!" There was a distant drone of an airplane engine, and we moved quickly across the highway. I did not want to be slimed with fire retardant.

Near the fire truck, I pulled on coveralls, boots and a water-filled backpack. I staggered off under the weight and began combing the bush for hotspots, watching a fellow volunteer dig at the ground with a long handled shovel. We fanned out towards the highway. The ground was full of forest debris, logs, fallen branches, stumps, bushes and uneven ground that kept tripping me. Every so often I would come across a blackened patch where fire had started, and I sprayed the spots down. The next few hours passed in a blur of sirens, water bombers, helicopters, smoke and exhaustion, and the forest fire was finally extinguished with no further damage to any homes or buildings in Robb.

"Robb Fire Department Responds to 10 Hectare Fire," the newspaper caption read.

"Fourteen fire fighters, operating a pumper, tanker and rescue responded. The forest fire was crowning in pine; it was estimated to be 100 feet above the tops of the trees. Forestry dispatched aircraft, the local emergency communication centre dispatched pumper trucks and tankers from surrounding communities, and members of the Robb community provided quads, trikes, manpower and refreshments. The fire originated from a coal seam fire at an abandoned coal mine."

I fell into bed that night and slept for over ten hours.

It was a dramatic start to the season, but reminded me that life is full of surprises and odd twists in the road. It was like Dad's open-heart surgery, which happened so fast we did not have time to think much about the pros and cons, implications and outcomes.

"Hi-ya, Kath, the surgery was successful," my father croaked into the phone late in May. "Everything's looking the way it's supposed to." What a relief! Dad would have another chance at continuing retirement life in Vancouver. I wished we lived closer but I had to be satisfied with phone calls and letters for now.

The summer flew by in a whirlwind of camping fees, firewood, dust, toilet paper, driving and more dust. The weather was good and campers came in droves on the holiday weekends. It was so encouraging, despite the endless work and the cost of operating campgrounds so far from services that most people took for granted, such as grocery stores and gas stations. Dave was exhausted, I was exhausted, and our kids were exhausted. After all that hard work we barely broke even. I almost cried.

At the general store in Robb at the beginning of September, I spotted an ad for a part-time teacher assistant at the local school. I immediately applied. The Robb Ranger Station was defunct and the guardian job that I had been doing since 1988 was obsolete. Our business generated very little income in the winter months, and even though Dave was sceptical about the plan, I felt I could handle the responsibilities. I would find a baby-sitter for Becky, which would help Dave to concentrate on new schemes for his campground business.

The aide job was to care for a special needs student three hours a day in the afternoon, and required someone physically fit with first aid experience. I could do that! Even if I was not sure about being in a room full of kids, I could take care of one child.

I got the job, and entered into a world of children that would steal my heart, teach me many valuable lessons, and send my life along different path.

THREE

"A child, more than all other gifts,
brings hope with it, and
forward-looking thoughts."
~ William Wordsworth ~

Working in an elementary school was not quite what I had expected. To me, kids meant noise, chaos and endless demands, but the quiet orderly routine dispelled any myths I may have held. It helped that the boy I worked with needed individualized care and attention, although I quickly became comfortable with children sharing our little space. No pretences were allowed. The kids and especially Steven helped me form a new perspective. He had cerebral palsy and communicated through his own world of sounds and limited upper-body motor control. Interpretation, instinct and compassion were part of the job of assisting a boy who was trapped inside his body and mind, slave to genetic malfunction and misfired neurons. Steven was tube fed, in diapers, in a wheelchair, and physically small. A specialty "seatbelt" kept him securely in place, pulling his shoulders back and preventing any surprise slides out of the chair. Lifting him in and out of the wheelchair was a challenge, especially as he grew.

A school field trip was planned that involved walking a kilometre to a pond on the outskirts of town, adjacent to the highway. It was a warm fall day and we decided

Steven would benefit from fresh air and an outing with fellow students. The kids crowded around his wheelchair.

"How come Steven doesn't talk?" one child asked. I paused before replying.

"He's not able to but he uses his eyes, funny sounds, and waves his arms to communicate. See, he's trying to grab your arm. Why don't you take his hand and say hi?" Most of the students accepted Steven's presence. Some even welcomed and included him in as many activities as possible. A few ignored him. I quickly learned how to engage the kids in responding to Steven and we made wonderful progress until Steven got sick. Then I fell and sprained my ankle, and we both missed some classroom time.

"I don't know how I managed to trip over my own feet," I said to the doctor as she gently pressed on my ankle.

"Ouch, it's sore!" I cried, looking down at the ugly purple bruising.

"Can you put any weight on it?" I stood up and gingerly tested it, surprised I could still bear my own weight. As soon as I moved, a sharp pain shot up my leg.

"I don't think it's broken. You need to stay off it for a few days until the swelling goes down. A tensor bandage and ice packs will help as well. Come back and see me if you have any problems."

A week later, I returned to the medical clinic.

"My ankle healed very quickly considering how hard I fell. You know, I'm not depressed any more. I'm feeling positive, focused and healthy; but the tiredness hasn't gone away. Without any reason or warning my legs just gave out last week when I sprained my ankle." I frowned and looked inquiringly at the doctor.

"Put one of these gowns on and I'll be right back." She closed the door behind her and soon returned with a little black case.

"Hop up on here." She tapped each knee with a funny rubber tool that looked like a hammer. "Lie down, please." The doctor opened the case and took out a fine bristled brush, which she ran down each leg and ended by tickling the bottom of my feet.

"Is this supposed to be funny?" I asked as she did the same thing with several different brushes and instruments from the mysterious black case. She smiled.

"You can get dressed now. I'll see you in a few minutes." I scrambled to put my clothes on, left the gown in a heap on the cold table, and retreated to a chair. There was a brief knock and the doctor entered.

"Kathy, this is a referral to see a specialist in Edmonton. It's a bit odd that you fell for no reason, and the chronic tiredness you mention is puzzling. I think further evaluation is necessary. Someone will call you to schedule an appointment."

"What kind of specialist?" I asked.

"A neurologist." I made a mental note to go to the library.

"What's that?"

"A neurologist specializes in the brain and central nervous system."

"Oh." I definitely needed to learn more.

~~~~~~

My oldest daughter Rachel was in grade six when I started working at the Bryan School in Robb. I looked forward to seeing her each day because I knew the following year she would ride the school bus sixty kilometres to Edson with the older kids to go to junior high and I would see much less of her. Rachel had been walking through the doors of the tiny school since

45

kindergarten, like many children before her, and was looking forward to a change. My friend, Bernadette, had taught Rachel in the early grades, and when circumstances took her to Edson, we remained friends despite the distance.

Enrolment in the Bryan School was dangerously low the autumn I began working as a teacher assistant. There were twenty-one students. Five students (one my own) would move on to attend junior high in Edson, an hour's drive away, the following year. With only sixteen remaining students, we were told it was economically unfeasible for the school to continue operating. We had reached the end of the road.

As a parent and an employee, I had a double interest in the fate of the Bryan School, which had been operating in Robb since 1951. A meeting was held in Edson to discuss the future of the school. Current teaching staff, interested parents, school board members and the school superintendent attended.

The statistics were not encouraging. Five-year projections for enrolment dropped below fifteen students, and with too many uncertain variables, it was apparent that the school division could not afford to keep the school open. Parents proposed fundraisers and teachers offered to juggle numbers for the school budget to see what costs could be cut in order to save money. The short-term solution bought another year.

I thought about our three-year old. In two years, Becky would be old enough to start kindergarten. Would we be willing to put her on a school bus at 7 am for the hour-long bus ride to Edson each day, to arrive home at 4.30 pm? Older children in the community had been doing this for years without too much difficulty and I knew Rachel would adapt, but it would be difficult for families with young children. There were options, but to me the future looked bleak.

Dave cut firewood that fall on his own. He went out into the bush a few times with neighbours who also needed wood, and hauled some excess from the campground. I was preoccupied with the kids, my father's failing health, my new job and my own mysterious health issues. Dave concentrated on making the business successful and all his projects, plans and schemes revolved around campgrounds. We were on different paths and could not seem to agree on anything.

Several times a month, Dave had been seeing a psychologist and we had tried several of her suggestions in an attempt to get our marriage back on track. One of the ideas was to spend some time together without the kids, job worries or any other distractions. It made me realize that all we ever did was work. Any recreation we did was tied to the business. We did not laugh; neither did we have fun. Conversations went round in circles until one day we found a common denominator: we both loved travelling.

Given our limited budget and time, we decided to explore locally and combine hostel and hotel accommodation. Dave liked hostels, and I had never had the opportunity to try the user-friendly, affordable option. We consciously tried to re-establish some intimacy and called a truce to our childish fighting. The trip was enjoyable. Perhaps it was possible to make this work after all.

The teachers were planning another outing for the students and they decided to take advantage of the school's proximity to the outdoor skating rink. We could see the shimmering ice from the classroom windows.

"Do you think Steven could come with us to the rink

if it's not too cold tomorrow?" Steven's teacher asked. "His mom said he has a sleigh at home they pull him around on sometimes. Maybe we could borrow it."

"I'll check with Dawn and see what we can arrange. I think Steven would like that."

I hoisted Steven out of his wheelchair onto my lap and grabbed the book we were going to look at during "silent reading." His right hand shot out enthusiastically to help turn the page. I gently guided his fingers that had difficulty with fine motor control and while he focused on the images, I whispered the words and prevented his hand from flipping the pages randomly.

After a few minutes, Steven's attention wandered and he looked around the classroom. Some heads were bent intently over an open book while others students flipped pages restlessly and made numerous trips to the bookstand, not really interested in the written word. Steven's head drooped. I switched to a brightly coloured hardcover book with large simple pictures. He wanted to touch the paper and feel with his fingers, a tactile movement that I had to monitor because his jerky reflexes sometimes ripped pages. Using cloth or stiff cardboard books helped.

The following afternoon, the weather was ideal for Steven and his classmates to be outside.

"Did you bring your skates, Kathy?" Steven's mother joked.

"I used to love skating, but I think I'll stick to 'terra firma' today, thanks." We both knew lifting and pulling Steven's seventy-pound frame was enough of a challenge without adding skates. The sun was shining and the air was still, crisp and clear. The rink had a thick layer of ice built up and the surface was smooth and glistening, a vast improvement over the bumpy uneven surface of a few years ago.

I had renewed my passion for figure skates and ice one day several years before when I took Rachel to the rink to teach her how to skate. Although I had started out wobbly and shaky, I was soon confidently skating laps. I used borrowed skates several more times, and then bought my own and began to skate whenever I had the chance. I had had some lessons as a kid and had tossed around a hockey puck with my brothers.

Rachel's feet hurt at first so she pushed an old chair around for support until she was able to stand on her own. When Rachel was tired I pushed while she sat. When the community added lights, we could skate at night. I had reached a point of gaining speed, strength, and learned to skate backwards.

My second pregnancy in 1994 had brought skating to a halt and I did not put on skates until a year later. The pleasure and excitement I had experienced was gone. My balance was off, my legs were like Jell-O, and I fell hard and often. I tried skating when I was well rested and energetic. I was still shaky and, unlike before, could not get past that point. By then Rachel did not need me with her because she had mastered staying upright on the ice and liked to skate with her friends. I stopped skating.

Egos are often fragile and mine was no exception. I was frustrated that I could not skate the way I used to. I was also confused and frustrated, blaming my lack of strength on having a baby at the age of thirty-five, denying that anything else could be wrong.

Steven loved the toboggan and being outdoors with his classmates. He wore a winter coat with a hood, insulated pants, boots, hat, mitts and a big smile. The wooden sleigh had curved rails; it was packed with padding and blankets. The first time I pulled the sleigh through soft snow with Steven strapped snugly on board, he let out a high-pitched squeal that turned to peals of laughter. The kids wanted to pull him and as soon as I was sure he was comfortably safe, I shared the joy of that magical afternoon with all who wanted to participate. Back and forth across the rink, with boundless energy, the kids pulled Steven until it was time to go home.

~~~~~~

I phoned my father in November. "This teacher assistant job is so amazing, Dad! After all those years of working for Forestry, being independent and on my own a lot, I figured I needed space and quiet to accomplish my tasks. This job is a lot different, but rewarding and challenging too." Dad listened patiently as I rambled on with some funny classroom stories. I suddenly remembered my father was facing his own challenges and quickly switched the subject. "What's new with you? How are plans coming for your birthday celebration in January?" Dad was turning seventy in the New Year. Becky and I were flying to Vancouver for a week, which I was really looking forward to.

"You know, Kathy, how I felt so good after my surgery in May and began walking and swimming to build up my strength? Well, something went screwy in about September and all my newfound energy was gone. I started feeling quite sick. After more poking prodding, numerous tests and waiting, the doctors determined the surgery hadn't fixed the problem I was having before, so I'm feeling a bit frustrated." His voice trailed off.

I took a deep breath. "You're kidding, right? That sounds completely unexpected. No wonder you're frustrated. Do the doctors have any idea what to do about this?"

"I have some new medication and they're monitoring

me closely, but our travel plans are on hold until we figure this thing out." Thank goodness he had his second wife, Pat, to care for him and help him through this.

"Okay, keep me posted. Love you." I hung up the phone. The news was unsettling, and I went outside in the frigid cold to split firewood while I mulled over what my father had told me. Please God, he has been through so much and waited so long for the surgery, help us to figure out what to do now to help.

At school, the students had begun planning a Christmas concert for the community and decided to have three short plays. The first one included all students, as well as various solo and group performances of piano, singing and dancing. Steven was nine years old, in grade three, and I expected he would be in the first play. I was surprised to learn he had never been in a Christmas concert before.

"It wouldn't be that hard to include him," I said. His teacher thought it was a great idea, his mother approved, and we started rehearsing for "How the Grump and the Grouch Stole Christmas." Steven was a "robin" along with a number of his classmates, and it was their job to flutter around the Christmas tree in excitement when the presents were stolen. We decided the kids could push Steven in his wheel chair and he would blend in with the commotion.

There were four narrow stairs leading up to the stage on either side, and getting Steven's wheelchair up those stairs was a chore. Lifting Steven up took all the strength I could muster, but it was worth the effort. Steven jammed his hand in his mouth and laughed his special laugh. I took that as approval. If his good health could only last until the night of the concert, we could follow through with our plan although I knew he was medically fragile and often missed school because of it, even ending up in the hospital. We could only try.

Dave and I were not communicating well again. I sensed his disapproval of my job commitment even though he was free to work on any project he chose, usually business related. We rarely had customers in the winter. The more time we spent together, the more we fought. I had hoped the short time spent apart would help our relationship; instead, it sparked more resentment. In fact, we were barely speaking.

I had scheduled a day off work to drive to Edmonton for the long awaited neurologist appointment in the busy month of December. I never made it out of the driveway.

Fighting broke out in the bedroom. Our own private war with weapons of the tongue caused irreversible damage. We argued and fought long into the night, resolving nothing and fuelling more bitterness and resentment. I pleaded exhaustion, insanity, and lost any ability to think clearly. Dave refused to let any of it go. The little things, the big stuff and everything in between were rehashed, including incidents that went back many years and had nothing to do with present circumstances. In my battle-weary state, I was unable to drive early the next morning. I dragged myself through the day in a state of confusion, hating myself for once again taking part in yet another useless fight and becoming the kind of person I despised - confrontational, angry, making a big deal out of nothing, and a drag to be around. I felt defeated and scared.

Dave announced he was leaving, was not sure where he was going, and didn't know if or when he was coming back. Before I had time to process his announcement, he was gone. I was relieved and secretly hoped he would not come back. The fighting had become intolerable. We had said and done terrible, hurtful things to each other that could never be taken back. I was so tired of the anger.

The girls and I carried on with our routine and Rachel did not question her father's sudden departure. No doubt she had heard plenty of arguments and sensed unhappiness in the house. I rescheduled the missed appointment in the city and shoved that worry to the back of my mind, having plenty to do with the needs of two children, a part-time job, and a household to keep together in the middle of a cold Alberta winter.

The Bryan School Christmas Concert at the local community hall was packed with families and excitement because Santa always made an appearance at the end of the evening, bringing gifts for the kids. Steven's mother phoned to let me know her son would be able to attend. I was pleased but nervous about lifting Steven up and down the stairs. He seemed heavier each time, and when a parent offered to bring him on stage after I voiced my concerns, I jumped at the offer. The performances were entertaining, funny and full of little errors that made it all the more enjoyable, especially when the kids wheeled Steven around the tree and made him a special part of the play. It was a highlight for me. I was proud of Rachel too, who was a narrator and did a great job.

Dave phoned a few days after Christmas. His soul searching had led him to a 12-Step Program in Vancouver where he had spent some time with friends and visited his mother.

"This 12-Step Program is really helping me, Kathy. I have a book that I can continue to work in, on my own, and I plan to be home the first week of January. Is Rachel around? Can I talk to her?"

I was sceptical that any program could help at this point, but at least Dave sounded positive and willing to move forward. The seething anger was gone, for now. Dave's unexpected return raised immediate issues I had left unresolved. Becky and I were flying to Vancouver for my father's seventieth birthday, and I was unsure about leaving Rachel behind. Now her routine would remain undisrupted and she could go to school.

My fantasy about Dave never returning was just that, a fantasy that had no place in our lives. I considered packing up the two kids and leaving but the reality was impossible. I had nowhere to go and little money. I would stick it out.

Sitting on the bookshelf in our house was a Medical Handbook that was a bit dated but had been a good reference book for me for about ten years. It was a natural place to start speculating about various diseases and medical conditions. I started at the beginning of this A to Z guide and scanned all kinds of peculiar names, descriptions that soon had my head reeling with the variety of ailments known to humanity. It was simple to eliminate as I went along. I stopped at "Depression" and read with detached interest.

"Depression as an illness implies a considerable and persisting change of mood, out of all proportion to the factors that may have triggered it off."

I thought about my visit to the doctor the previous year when she told me I was probably depressed, the recognition that I was not feeling well or my usual self, and how dramatically different I felt when the "fog" lifted after a few months. It was unfamiliar territory to me, although I was aware my mother, husband and a few friends had suffered periodically from this confusing disorder.

I spent several sessions with the book when I came to a disease called *"Multiple Sclerosis."* Multiple what?? I had never heard of it before but clearly identified with what it said. I read the description over several times and then broke it down into sections.

"A chronic disease of the central nervous system in which patches of defective and hardened tissue appear at random in the brain and spinal cord and interfere with the normal function of the affected parts. The condition is also called disseminated sclerosis. Its cause is unknown."

At this point, all I knew was the central nervous system included the brain and spinal cord. I read the next paragraph and my heart gave a jolt.

"The disease usually starts at twenty to forty years (practically never after fifty), and its course is progressive with increasing disability, although temporary remissions are a feature. The typical symptoms are weakness, lack of coordination, rigidity and paralysis of the lower limbs (spastic paraplegia) together with the very characteristic and often associated occurrence of nystagmus, tremor of the arms, and a peculiar scanning or syllabic speech."

I was thirty-nine, and had experienced unexplained weakness, lack of coordination and rigidity, a different word for stiffness, and more tiredness than I had ever felt in my life. The paralysis and tremor did not apply to me, thank God, but the parallels to the rest of the symptoms listed could not be denied. Fortunately, the last paragraph, which mentioned the lack of treatment available, did not enter into my realm of thinking at the time and, as I found out later, was outdated.

I needed plenty of time to think things through and I carried on after my little discovery without much concern. There was no personal experience to base it on and even after reading more about MS at the local library and talking to a few trusted friends, I really had no idea of the implications of such a diagnosis. Maybe it was something else, anyway, something not listed in the book. "Take one step at a time," I told myself.

Dave was a different person when he returned. I was confused. He had left so full of anger but returned mellow and positive, attributing his newfound outlook to the 12-Step Program. Through my attendance at Al-Anon, my brother's participation in a Narcotics Anonymous Program, and my mother's short stint in A.A. many years earlier, I was aware of the life saving nature of these types of programs, so I accepted the sincere effort Dave was making. We attended a couple of marriage counselling sessions through a local organization that only served to confuse my recognition that our relationship was in serious jeopardy. Travel distance, cost and lack of understanding on my part of the role I played kept us from continuing this route. All I did was cry. The façade of a positive atmosphere in our home soon changed back to negative, and I felt trapped in gloom.

~~~~~~

"Well, Becky, this is your first plane ride," I said to my three-year old daughter as the plane took off.

"Good afternoon, passengers. This is your captain speaking on behalf of Air Canada Flight 148 to Vancouver. Today we'll be cruising at an altitude of 32,000 feet with a flying time of 1 hour and 30 minutes. In case of any turbulence, please keep your seatbelts fastened." I was looking forward to the break in usual routine, and spending time with Dad.

Mike warned me how thin Dad had become but my brother could not have prepared me for the skeleton of a man that greeted us. I probably hugged him too hard and tried not to stare. Becky was a good distraction.

There were no long walks or big outings on this trip because it was obvious Dad was not well, but his birthday celebration at a favourite restaurant with a dozen or so family members was wonderful. My own health concerns were pushed aside, overshadowed by my father's deteriorating condition.

My appointment to see a neurologist at the end of January was brief and to the point. After a physical examination, I asked him what he thought it might be.

"I can't be certain until we do more tests," he said guardedly. I stared him down.

"Could it be multiple sclerosis?" I asked, my tongue fumbling over the words. The doctor hesitated.

"We need to rule out a number of other possibilities before making any clear diagnosis. I'd like to schedule you for an MRI, VER and SER. After that, we should be able to determine more. Someone will call you with the appointment dates."

"What are VER and SER?" I asked nervously. The doctor actually smiled.

"The ER stands for evoked response, which is a measurement of nerve conduction. A few electrodes are taped to different parts of your body as the test is done. It doesn't take long or hurt at all."

I filed the new information away along with the letter that arrived a few weeks later summarizing the initial visit.

"On neurological examination, mental status and cranial nerves are unremarkable." In layman's terms, this meant he couldn't find anything wrong.

"Strength is five out of five and actually is considerably above normal in every muscle tested." I read this over several times to reassure myself. "Reflexes are brisk and she has sustained clonus on the left. Plantars are down going. Both legs are mildly spastic." That did not sound good. "She has moderate loss of vibratory sense. Pinprick and light touch are unremarkable. Tests of coordination are unremarkable. Her tandem gait is minimally off especially for her athletic abilities. Having her do rapid squats, she did thirty without a problem. I retested her strength and it was the same."

I thought I was still strong, but now I had confirmation. Just this crazy tiredness needed to be addressed.

Al-Anon was teaching me about powerlessness and how to "Let go, and let God." It applied to so many things that I had no control over in my life. I could control my health by making good choices, but after that, it was not up to me. I could control my actions, my words, but after that, I could not change others. Going to the meetings was helping me get a sense of myself. It brought some healing and self-forgiveness. I had a glimpse of the suffering my alcoholic mother must have gone through and a better understanding of how much I was affected by her behaviour and attitudes. The power to change - that was going to be the hard part.

FOUR

"If Anything Can Go Wrong, It Will."
~ Murphy's Law ~

I spent time over Christmas researching the local job market in the nearby communities of Jasper, Hinton and Edson. Dave had said he might not be back, and I was tired of the restrictions and isolation I felt living in Robb. I made some inquiries about types of jobs available in Jasper National Park. When a Park official outlined a job description of long hours and heavy manual labour in the campgrounds, I said I had plenty of experience, which was true but what was I thinking? I was exhausted when I least expected to be, despite what the doctor said about my strength, and had two kids to care for as well. It was discouraging but a good reality check, and when Dave came home in January, I shelved the whole idea as impossible.

Steven was sick on and off in January and February and the teachers kept me busy with odd jobs until there were no more and I had a few weeks off. We tried some home visits to keep Steven's routine going, but it was not the same as being in the classroom with the other children and eventually we gave up this approach.

A teacher assistant conference in Edmonton provided me with some new ideas, as did accompanying Steven on his annual visit to see a variety of specialists at the Glenrose Rehabilitation Hospital. This trip was valuable in providing insight into Steven's particular needs and continued development and I became familiar with terms and jargon used to follow his condition. It allowed me to develop a report card specific to Steven's special needs and aided in setting realistic goals. The goals were simple things like "four out of five times Steven will reach for a named object," but very useful in determining his understanding and building on that.

Steven was, at the best of times, very shaky as part of the cerebral palsy, which was controlled heavily with medication. One day, he was shaking violently no matter what I tried.

"Hi Dawn. Steven is having a rough day. I think it would be better if he went home. He can't stop shaking and has pooped his pants twice. I've never seen him like this." I pulled Steven into my lap and held him tightly in an attempt to still the tremors that shook his body, but the trembling continued. I felt helpless. It was impossible to follow our usual routine and Steven became more upset as time progressed, so when his mother arrived to take him home, I was relieved. I hoped he was not getting sick again.

It was sunny and mild in April when I drove to Edmonton for my "evoked response" testing and I turned up the music and sang along in an off-key voice, happy to be by myself. Heading eastward along Highway 16, also known as Death Highway before a twinning expansion in about 1990, I glanced in the rear-view mirror at the snow-capped peaks of the Rocky Mountains that covered the western horizon. The massive, shaved rock, with the odd rounded top and a tree line of coniferous pine and spruce, included Jasper and Banff National Parks, where I had enjoyed downhill and cross-country skiing, as well as many memorable hikes. Rocky Mountain bighorn sheep with their scruffy greyish fur and large curly horns were often seen along the highway and majestic brown and tan-coloured elk roamed the grassy low-lying fields around Jasper.

As I drove east, the mountains changed into foothills and it was not uncommon to see white-tailed or mule deer, moose or a coyote in the ditch. What would happen if I hit one of these animals? I had heard plenty of scary stories, but my fears proved unfounded. Wildlife flourished despite the hazards of man and nature.

The ponds and lakes that dotted the landscape remained frozen. As I drove eastward, the land flattened out to undulating hills and soon agricultural land predominated. Cattle, horses, wheat and canola fields caught my eye. Deciduous trees stood stark, awaiting the miracle of spring after a long harsh winter of dormancy. In the summer the wet, slushy ditches would dry up and become a sea of tall grass, daisies and fireweed. Three hundred kilometres later, I was in West Edmonton for the required medical tests.

"Wait here and someone will be with you in a minute," the woman in the white lab coat said politely. Soon, another technician was taping electrodes to my head.

"Sit as still as you can, please. It will take about ten minutes, and you'll feel some pulsing and vibrations on your skin while the machine is running." The electrodes were moved to my arms, and then several locations on my legs and feet, and ten minutes turned into an hour. The doctor was right; it did not hurt but it was an unusual sensory experience. Sometimes it tickled, felt heavy, vibrated lightly or intensely on the skin – almost prickly, then oddly numbing, or I felt nothing at all.

"What did you find?" I asked when it was finished.

"We'll send the results to your doctor and he or she will talk to you about it," came the automatic response.

More waiting; more testing. The MRI (magnetic resonance imaging) was scheduled at the university hospital in early June.

~~~~~~

Dave and I did not renew the contract to operate Fairfax Lake for the summer of 1998. I had hoped the expansion would tip the scales towards profit but the cost to operate had gone up significantly. Dave had hired a young man to help him and costs again exceeded the income. It was such a beautiful area but the remote location did not draw the number of customers needed to support the business. The people who came were mostly self-sufficient. It was the fourth year of operation.

Temperatures remained warm, and snow and ice disappeared quickly. The Fire Department decided to burn brush around town to speed the "green up" process and clear garbage that had accumulated around the school, park, hotel and ditches. At first, I thought it only created an ugly black mess, but with a little spring rain and sunshine, the grass and shrubs turned green quickly. The ground was cleared of debris. I looked forward to the event where volunteers split into smaller groups and only needed to wear bright orange coveralls, insulated boots, and helmets. Light joking and camaraderie prevailed as we practised and developed our skills using firefighting equipment. The early spring evening was calm and I forgot about my tiredness.

"Hey, Kathy, grab a rake and we'll make sure the flames don't go past the top of the hill," shouted a fellow firefighter. I started up the short slope, bent my head down to avoid branches poking me, and stumbled over a log on the ground. I lifted my head to regain my balance and a sharp branch brushed across my face. It stung and my eye watered. Dark smoke surrounded me, and I scrambled towards the road, coughing, and collapsed on the ground. Exhaustion set in as I dragged myself through the final controlled burn, impatient for the session to end.

The optometrist's voice interrupted my thoughts.

"There's a small scratch on the cornea which is causing the eye to weep. I've written you a prescription for an antibiotic to prevent infection, which you should start taking right away." I rubbed my eye hard. It was a minor injury but I was surprised how quickly it happened despite protective clothing.

The May "Victoria Day" long weekend was often the first busy weekend of the camping season, and we had been working hard to prepare. I helped purchase supplies and kept the books updated, but this year Dave would do most of the "hands-on" work himself. On the surface, our relationship was in neutral. For now, the roller coaster had levelled out.

Rachel was nearing the end of grade six, which meant she would ride the bus to Edson in the fall to attend junior high school.

"Mom, I've waited so long for this chance to start fresh and make some new friends. Getting up early will be hard but will be worth it! You should see the long hallways and the giant gymnasium they have. And the cafeteria is so cool."

"I can hardly wait for you to start, too, Rachel. Grade seven. It sounds so … grown-up." My daughter was tired of the limitations of a two-room schoolhouse with only five kids at her grade level.

"We're having a graduation ceremony right after the last achievement test and I'll be done grade six forever!" Rachel's eyes sparkled. The Bryan School had been granted one final year of operation and was slated to close, but Rachel did not mind. She was moving on to bigger and better things. I was saddened by the news of the school closing because it meant my job would end. I had come to love working in a school, but something else might happen to prevent or prolong the closure, and I was not going to dwell on that now.

Before the long weekend, I drove to Edson for last-minute supplies. The air was cool and little puffs of ground fog filled many of the dips. Upon approaching one such spot, I realized the ground fog was actually smoke, coming from the ditch right-of-way on the east side, where a vehicle was pulled off with the engine idling. Two guys leaned on the hood. My eyes followed some gouged out tracks in the wet muskeg down a bit of a slope, to find an overturned logging truck and logs spread haphazardly about. These massive trucks were a common sight on the local roads. I slowed down and rolled down the passenger window a few inches.

"What happened?"

"Logging truck went off the road. We radioed for help."

"Is anybody hurt?" The men looked blankly at me.

"The driver didn't make it." I swallowed hard and pulled over. As a firefighter with first aid training, I had a duty to check for myself. My legs shook as I stepped sideways down the hill towards to the truck. I could see logs had come straight through the cab, back to front. Some smoke was coming from under the hood and I peered closer to see a man's body lying in the wildly strewn logs. When I got close enough to touch him, I recoiled in horror. His injuries were beyond the scope of my imagination and I knew no amount of first aid could bring back this life. I dragged myself up the hill as our fire department's rescue van arrived and two fellow volunteers rushed down with a first aid kit and blankets. They returned for a body bag and I left the scene.

I went through the day like a zombie and drove slowly by the accident scene on the way home. One life had been lost so suddenly. There was barely any evidence of what had taken place except for the ruts in the muskeg, and I shivered. The scene played over and over in my mind for days. A few weeks later, I saw a wreath marking the spot where the driver had been killed and I was touched by this symbol of honour. A family was grieving.

It turned hot a few days before the holiday weekend and the long-range forecast was promising. Late on Monday afternoon the phone rang.

"Hi Kath, how are you?" Dad asked in a gravelly voice.

"Dad? Good to hear from you. I'm not bad, how's it going?" Dad's voice levelled out as he talked and I listened carefully as he spoke.

"I've been scheduled for surgery again ... on Wednesday. The doctors say it's my only hope now. I came through it before. We'll get through it this time, too." I could feel my heart beating faster.

"Does Mike know? How come they gave you such short notice?" I had a million questions as my mind started racing, but my voice remained calm.

"Mike will be there, Pat will be there, and they'll keep you posted." I smiled at his matter of fact tone.

"Okay, Dad, I'll be thinkin' about you and praying for the best. You take care." I was scared, but I am sure his fear far exceeded mine.

I talked to Mike on the phone and he assured me he would be at the hospital on Wednesday. I was grateful to be busy with the details of the business, my job and family. Even though concentrating was hard, at least it gave me some focus. The next day at work, I shared my fears with the two teachers I worked with.

"If you need to take some time off, Kathy, don't worry about your job. We'll hire someone if we need to. Steven will be fine." Their compassion was overwhelming, but I did not have a clear sense of what to do. How could I leave Dave to run the campground on his own on the first busy weekend of the season? What about my commitment to my daughters? But what about my father whom I loved so much, and my brother Mike who was also very close to Dad and sick with worry and fear? I felt torn and distraught.

I could do nothing except keep busy and play the waiting game, something I was good at. The day still dragged and I finally talked to Mike in the early evening.

"Yeah, he's still in recovery in intensive care. The important thing is that he wakes up in the next while. I'll call when I know more."

I talked to my Dad's wife, Pat, and my brother Paul. It was too soon to know very much, except that Dad had made it through a second open-heart surgery within a year of the first. I focused on that fact, because I knew the odds were not in his favour, especially at seventy years of age and in deteriorating health. Only a small percentage of patients in his circumstances made it out of the hospital. It was a grim statistic.

Over the next twenty-four hours, I talked to Mike several times. Dad was hanging on by a thread and the doctors were not optimistic. After a disturbed and restless sleep on Thursday night, I went to work on Friday afternoon with a heavy heart. I listened to my colleague's encouragement, opinions and ideas and it was suddenly clear what needed to be done. I could take the girls with me. Within twenty-four hours, Rachel, Becky and I were walking in the door of my brother's home in Vancouver.

Mike took me to the hospital where Dad lay hooked up to monitors and tubes, in a darkened sterile room with others who lay still and unconscious as they struggled to overcome the trauma of surgery. A few of the beds were empty. Machines whirred, beeped and flashed in a crazy kaleidoscope of unfamiliar patterns, and Mike and I automatically spoke in hushed tones.

"He looks so pale and sick," I whispered as my voice broke. My eyes remained dry. Mike stared at one of the screens for a minute.

"You know what, Kath, he's doing a lot better than yesterday even though it's still a critical-care scenario." Mike looked around the large room at other patients lying mute with life support aiding each laboured breath. "I've been told a lot of patients never make it out of this room. The most important thing now is that Dad wakes up within ten days of the surgery, or the odds for his recovery are very low."

I went and held Dad's hand because it was the only thing free of tubes and equipment. It was cool and still, unresponsive to my gentle squeeze.

"I got a hold of some of Dad's favourite music and it will be played on and off. He can have visitors, only family, and for very short periods. Pat and her family will come too, so he'll have company every day. That's about all we can do."

"Has Paul been in yet?" I asked. The middle child with his own set of problems, Paul was a workaholic who did not like hospitals or family commitments. Mike frowned.

"Once, I think. A friend came with him. He was pretty freaked out."

"Maybe we can meet at the hospital while I'm here," I said, always willing to try to include our elusive brother in our plans. Paul and I had not done anything more than have a meal together in years, so I tried to keep my expectations low.

A nurse came in to check the dressing on Dad's incision. We decided it was a good time to leave. I would come back tomorrow, perhaps on my own.

I placed my confidence in my father's strong will to live, competent doctors, current medical technology and faith that it was out of my hands. I recognized that it was beyond my control, which allowed me to concentrate on my role. I took my daughters to see their Grandpa, went alone, met with Paul at Dad's bedside, and met Pat and her family. We never gave up hope that he would recover, even though nine days had passed since the surgery. Friday was my last day to visit, as the girls and I needed to journey home to Alberta.

Sometime between Thursday and Friday, Dad woke up. He was moved out of intensive care! We were all so excited, and when I arrived, Dad was semi-sitting in bed eating ice chips. I told him we had been in Vancouver for a week and that we were driving back to Alberta the following day.

"It's a long drive," he croaked, and I was elated his memory was clear and that we could return home with our hopes buoyed.

~~~~~~

Thick, lush coastal vegetation slowly changed to spacious, arid, interior scrubland as we climbed through mountain ranges, towns and villages from sea level to over three thousand feet. North of Kamloops the forests grew dense again as we left ponderosa pine and brown sage brush behind, and enjoyed a brief drive along the lazy Clearwater River with its characteristic rich green grasses and graceful weeping willows. Long, agricultural sprinklers kept the ground saturated and further along, farm animals and old barns dotted the open fields. We drove higher and along the mighty Fraser River. The drive went on and on northward through mountains and valleys, until we finally turned east and headed through Mount Robson National Park. The park was a rugged outdoorsman's dream, filled with magnificent forests, lakes and spectacular peaks that sat adjacent to the Alberta border and Jasper National Park. Only a couple of hours drive remained for us.

The Rocky Mountains dominated the landscape, adding depth and beauty to the remaining drive. I tried to appreciate the wondrous scenery but tiredness settled upon me..

"Mom, it's taking forever," Rachel said as I handed her a pack of gum. Becky was asleep in her car seat.

"Rachel, you know how close we're getting, and you won't have to travel again for a while." I carefully gripped the wheel over the last fifty kilometres of dusty gravel in the dusk of late evening. Several white-tailed deer crossed our path and kept me alert for the unexpected.

At least I had a chance to get into a regular routine before travelling to Edmonton for an MRI. The University Hospital was a three-hour drive east. I felt as though we lived far, far away from anywhere.

~~~~~~

Upon entry, the hospital was alive with activity. A huge, bright atrium filled with plants and a trickling fountain belied the Spartan, sterile rooms beyond. I was soon lost in a maze of hallways and doors that seemed to go on forever, with people in uniforms rushing by and disappearing mysteriously. I felt a bit like Alice in Wonderland. I stopped several times to check the map (I always read maps) and eventually ended up in the lobby of diagnostic imaging. It was packed. Some emergencies had disrupted the schedule and my appointment was delayed by several hours. It was not common, I was told. I found my way back to the main entrance and wandered the strip of eateries and gift shops before riding the glass-encased elevator many floors above. The hospital was a place of beauty, sadness and healing. The miracle of life began and ended here. I stopped for some food and slowly made my way back to the waiting room.

"Here's some earplugs for you to wear while you're being tested," the person in the white lab coat said.

"Will it take long?"

"About an hour. Are you claustrophobic at all?" I actually thought it was kind of cool.

"Not at all." The lab technician directed me to lie down and cocooned my head and body in hardware needed for the imaging. He placed a plastic emergency buzzer in my hand in case of any problems.

"You need to lie as still as you can. There's a speaker in the tube so we can communicate with you and vice versa. Do you have any questions?" I shook my head. Suddenly the bed rolled backwards and I was swallowed in a tunnel-shaped hollow tube.

"Okay, Kathy? Are you comfortable?"

"Yes, fine." The headset was digging into my skull, but I would survive. When the sound effects started up, I forgot about everything else. *"Tap, tap, tap. Click. T–t-t-t-t-t-t-t"*. It was loud. The tapping in various patterns went on for several minutes. Ten seconds of silence preceded another barrage of strange sounds. I tried not to laugh. It sounded like machine guns, slow motion changing to rapid fire. Then silence.

"Kathy, we'd like you to try your best not to swallow for the next few minutes. Take a deep swallow now, and

70

we'll begin." It sounded so easy, but within forty-five seconds, I had the urge to swallow. No matter how hard I willed it to go away, the urge persisted and feeling like a failure, I gave up and took a careful swallow. I had no idea I swallowed so much. Gulp. It became the focal point, and suppressing my need to swallow made it worse. So much for relaxing! I swallowed again.

"How are you doin' in there, Kathy? We're finished in the neck area and moving onto the spine. There will be a series of new sounds that will last about seven minutes."

I swallowed several times in celebration, and had a new appreciation of my swallowing reflex.

"Whaaaaa, hahhhhh" went the machine in a deep, low-pitched baritone. I closed my eyes and imagined I was on a ship at sea, surrounded by ships sounding their horns. Big ships, little ships, a lighthouse, fog, and stormy weather became the backdrop for various "distress" horns. The visual was a perfect match for the sounds.

"Bump-bump-bump-bump-bump, honnnk, bang." My new location was a noisy construction site with the *"rat-a-tat-tat"* of a jackhammer and the *"tink, tink, tink"* of nails sinking into wood. There was no sleeping on this journey.

Just when I was getting tired of the whole process and felt the headpiece digging in, it ended. The strange noises stopped and the tube spat me out. The MRI was complete.

Mike phoned a few days later. He sighed heavily.

"Dad's had a setback, Kathy. He's picked up some kind of infection that's being treated with antibiotics, but so far nothing's working. Unfortunately he's been placed in isolation until this thing is under control."

"I don't know what to say. It's not fair. He was doing

so well when I left. Paul said he even pushed Dad around the hospital in a wheelchair and that he was happy and coherent." I hung up with a new set of worries.

I was travel weary and scheduled my appointment to meet with the neurologist at the end of June to get the results of the MRI. After all the months of waiting and wondering what was wrong, I suddenly had to know. The doctor returned my call that evening.

"Yes, the MRI shows abnormality in the brain and cervical cord. This is probable cause for multiple sclerosis. We can discuss the details when you come to the city for your appointment."

I was relieved. There was a name for this invisible monster inside of me that was stealing my energy and we would do whatever it took to combat the situation. Other than the energy drain, I was certainly not sick.

My Dad was the one who was ill and I worried more each time I talked to Mike or Pat. The infection was a "super bug," a bacterial strain highly resistant to drugs and especially dangerous to the young and elderly. This was way past "not fair." Now that I knew Dave could manage the business on his own, I decided another trip to the coast in July was critical. My father was not improving.

On June 30, 1998, I sat in the neurologist's office in Edmonton and listened impartially to his opinions and recommendations. The unfamiliar medical jargon served to buffer my fears and I thank God to this day for my ignorance about the disease and the implications it carried. Otherwise, I would have been devastated. The follow-up letter I received after the meeting recapped the neurologist's summary.

"The diagnosis at this time is probable MS and I have explained the nature of the disease with the aid of a pamphlet which I gave to her. She has the number and address of the MS Society for further information and support. She has a good understanding of the disease and a positive attitude."

I walked out into the warm, sunny day confidently. Adversity was no stranger to me. But the doctor had lied. I did not have a good understanding of MS. As I would learn, it is a fickle, silent invader, no friend of mine.

FIVE

"Whisper words of wisdom,
let it be, let it be."
~ The Beatles ~

"Dad is dying," I said to Dave as we discussed summer plans. "It's where I need to be. For years, I have wished we could spend more time together, but the distance has been too great and we have been so busy. I will take the kids and you'll have only yourself, the dog and the business to take care of. The paperwork can pile up and I'll take care of it when I get back."

Expressing thoughts about death did not make it seem any more real but I no longer felt torn between obligations. It might be my last chance to spend any time with Dad, even if it was in the hospital. Dave's mother lived in Vancouver and had offered us her place for two weeks while she travelled to Ontario. I gratefully accepted, knowing it would extend our stay and give us the freedom we needed. We planned to spend the first two weeks with friends and relatives.

Vancouver in the summer! I was excited. It was the first summer in years that I had not had to work and the girls shared in my enthusiasm.

"What will we do, Mom?" Rachel asked.

"Lots of things like going to the beach, parks, and exploring the city. We'll start out each day visiting Grandpa and then decide what we want to do. We'll stay with relatives until Grandma goes to Ontario, and then we can stay at her place. There's supposed to be a really spectacular fireworks display, Uncle Mike wants to take us on his boat, and Alison thought you might like Science World." Rachel was satisfied and I guessed she would not be bored in the city. It turned out to be a magical bonding time for the three of us.

The hospital was huge, bright and clinically clean, with hidden danger lurking in unsuspecting places that had put my Dad flat on his back, again. It smelled strongly of antiseptic. I walked down the long hallway that connected to the isolation care wing, and looked out the line of glass windows at the clear blue sky and coastal mountains. I glanced down at my shorts and sandaled feet that were in sharp contrast to hospital uniforms, and thought about the warmth of the sun and the lucky people walking around outside. We take health for granted until something goes wrong and we are forced to change our ways.

The nurse at the reception desk told me to wash my hands before donning the gown and gloves provided, as well as a mask that covered my mouth and nose. She gave me a pamphlet about Dad's condition, which I tucked away in my purse to look at later. I left my things outside the room and noticed a dark-haired woman sitting in a chair by the window.

"Who's that?" I asked, surprised.

"That's a lady from our hospital auxiliary who provides backup support to those who need it. Because a nurse can't stay with your father at all times, this group provides constant monitoring and basic care to supplement the professional care nurses and doctors provide. It's a twenty-four hour service. I think it's eight or twelve hour shifts."

"Wow, I didn't realize the extent of care involved."

"Your father's very sick. Are you ready to go in?" She smiled at me briefly. I adjusted the mask and took a deep breath.

"Okay, let's go."

Dad's eyes were closed. The bed was propped up slightly to a semi-sitting position, and I rushed over to stand beside him.

"Dad, it's Kath," I said in a whisper. His eyes opened in the thin, sunken face and his exposed arm was covered in bruises from various needles required over the past six weeks, I guessed. "You've got your own room this time, with a view of the mountains."

He stared at me as he reached out a hand to squeeze the mask covering my lower face. I could see some humour glimmering in those brilliant blue eyes, and I laughed.

"I know, it's like a duck's beak, but the doctors say we have to wear them. I can't even give you a kiss."

Dad smiled and I was sure he recognized me. He was not able to talk, but seemed eager to communicate, so I looked around for something for him to write on. The aide had taken a break during my visit so we were on our own. I spotted a red vinyl clipboard on the window ledge. Perfect. It was filled with lined paper and I handed it to Dad. He fumbled with positioning the pen and then began to write a jumble of words, with a diagram that made no sense. Disappointed, I pushed it aside and sat down. Dad's gaze shifted to the white ceiling tiles above that had rows and rows of endless dots, with their own special Braille-like pattern that kept Dad's eyes transfixed upward.

I stopped my nervous chatter and surveyed the isolation room. A hospital bed, side table, two chairs, a television and an empty window ledge filled the space along with a portable intravenous stand, aluminum walker, and wheelchair. A door stood ajar and revealed a large tiled bathroom. The only attractive sight was beyond the large picture window where tree-clad mountains stood in splendour. I would ask my daughters, niece and nephew to draw or colour some pictures to cheer the room up, and give Dad something other than dots on the ceiling to contemplate in his befuddled state.

The Father's Day card I had sent was nowhere in sight. I searched through the red clipboard carefully for the photocopy of the short story I had tucked inside the card and had asked Pat to read aloud to my father. It was called "Pedal" and I thought it was an encouraging message to "hang in there." The reader was told to give God the front seat of the tandem bicycle, the control part, and to simply trust, give and receive, and best of all, hang on and enjoy the ride "through long cuts, up mountains, through rocky places and at breakneck speeds." Dad had encouraged me for most of my life, and it was my turn to help him find hope.

Later on that evening, I pulled out the pamphlet the nurse had given me. "MRSA," it said. *Methicillin resistant staphylococcus aureus,* a bacterial super bug, resistant to many antibiotics, that commonly infects hospital patients but rarely infects healthy people. A bacterium found on the skin, which can get into the body through wounds and needles. The pamphlet noted the importance of vigilant hygiene: hand-washing, gloving, masking, gowning, sterilizing and disinfecting equipment.

Through the media, I understood super bugs were difficult to treat but I refused to think the worst. Dad's will to live was strong.

The weather was beautiful. After visiting my Dad each day, the girls and I explored parks, beaches, stores and restaurants. Neighbourhood parks were set up with family fun in mind because many had jetted water park areas creatively arranged, with bright metal sprinklers of various shapes and sizes so that kids and parents alike ran through screaming, laughing, and gasping in the summer halo of heat. It was unusually hot for the West Coast but we did not complain.

We made a memorable trip to Stanley Park, located on the west side of the city near the downtown core. It contained lovely beaches, a long seawall walkway, old growth forests of cedar, maple and Douglas fir, an aquarium, zoo, and miniature train. Ponds, birds and lush coastal growth surrounded us as we wandered around. Squawking gulls and bird poop were minor hazards in this lotus land that sat beside the Pacific Ocean.

I knew why my father loved Vancouver. Even in the winter with never-ending rain and fog, one sunny day instantly dispelled the gloom. I felt blessed to be able to show my kids the city where I grew up at its best and they rarely complained of the hospital trips because they knew something interesting was in store afterwards.

One day we discovered an RV park/campground on the North Shore, beside the ocean, that had a small tenting area underneath the Lions Gate Bridge. It was directly across the water from Stanley Park. We had already slept comfortably in our SUV on the trip from Alberta. With warm weather, we decided a few days of camping might be fun. It was surprisingly quiet given all the traffic passing over us.

"Let's walk across the bridge," I suggested, with an eye for adventure. A set of stairs led up to the bridge walkway from the south end of the campground. I had driven, walked and biked across the picturesque bridge many times in the past.

"There will be a lot of cars, so we need to stay on the sidewalk and be careful." Rachel nodded and I held Becky's hand tightly.

"It's noisy, mom." Rachel covered her ears.

"Plug your nose, too," I warned as the stench of vehicle fumes hit me.

To the east, Burrard Inlet was home to many docks, boats and seaside activity as well as the north edge of downtown, where the white wings of Canada Place dominated. The west opened up to a larger expanse of Pacific Ocean as ferries, ships, sailboats and motorboats shared the water, while glimpses of land that were part of the Gulf Islands composed the background. The water sparkled and a ship's horn sounded. A light breeze carried pungent ocean smells of seaweed and salt.

I shielded Becky's small frame from the vehicles driving by and we stopped several times to survey the scene. The suspension bridge shook.

"Mom, can we go back?" Rachel yelled. Traffic shot by.

"Sure. It's loud, huh?"

"It's the shaking that's bothering me. I don't feel safe." We turned around and headed back, where beyond the bridge and immediate mountains the double-peaked "Lions" stood tall in the distance.

Years before, I rode across the bridge on my bicycle without a second thought, the traffic and noise barely registering on my consciousness, muscles taut, eyes sharp and mind conditioned to the multi-use of space. It was strange how twenty years (and probably increased traffic) could change one's perspective!

The days blended into one another like an artist's watercolour painting. Beautiful colours, vibrant scenery and an eclectic mix of people and cultures were stimulating. We were caught up in the faster pace of a more varied lifestyle, but I did not feel stressed because of it. Certainly, there were many more people than we were used to. Line-ups and traffic were everywhere, but because I was not working, we could usually avoid the busier times of day for most of our needs.

By the middle of July, we were settled in North Vancouver, in the girls' grandmother's condominium. At this time, my father experienced yet another setback in his health. Mike phoned me early one evening.

"Dad had a tracheotomy today, Kathy. He was having so much trouble breathing he started choking. With a trach, the congestion in his lungs can be dealt with. I think there's also a catheter, as he's being given steady liquids." Mike sighed. I coughed back my guilt.

"I haven't been in for a couple of days. It's kind of far from North Van and the last time we went, Dad didn't wake up, and it seemed so pointless. We had a good visit about a week ago and I felt encouraged but all the days following, he was unresponsive. I'll go tomorrow. Have you been in?"

"No, I've been working a lot. There was a message on our voice mail when I got in. I'll swing by the hospital later." Mike lived in the area.

"I'll call Paul if you want."

"Okay. Talk to you later." The phone clicked.

I anxiously set my alarm clock that night and rolled around restlessly in the hot room. The heat wave was oppressive.

I left the girls in the hospital cafeteria eating cubes of slippery green Jell-O with whipped cream. Familiar food odours did not disguise the pervasive, lingering hospital smells I encountered as I made my way to the fifth floor. Nearing the isolation wing, I slowed my pace

80

and peered curiously into the hospital rooms. Bed after bed, patient after patient, machine after machine, it was a sea of illness. There were many elderly patients, a few moving about, but most still with eyes closed or staring straight ahead. I shuddered. It seemed like such a sad, lonely place.

As I donned the all-too-familiar mask and gown, I looked through the glass at the figure lying on the bed. There was some new equipment surrounding Dad, and I took a deep breath before I entered.

If Dad could possibly have been thinner, he was thinner. The trach tube snaked its way from a hole in his throat to a machine. It was unnatural but it was helping him stay alive, so I focused on his eyes and tried not to look at the traces of blood on his neck, the bruises on his arms and the catheter bag hanging half covered off the side of the bed.

"Hi, Dad." His eyes were vacant. "They've sure got you fixed up here. Guess you won't be doing any night-time jogs." He stared upward and I turned my head to hide sudden watery eyes.

Each visit was similar. Dad was either sleeping or staring. One day the nurse came in to suction off the phlegm in his lungs that made his breathing so difficult.

"How often is this done?" I asked as the nurse hooked up the suction tube.

"Pardon?" she said, as the noisy procedure drowned out any speech and Dad's face contorted. Nauseous fumes permeated my mask.

"Every few hours or as often as needed to improve Len's breathing."

"What about his medication? How's that going?" The nurse grabbed a clipboard hanging on the wall.

"He's on a new round of antibiotics and it's too soon to tell if anything is changing."

The first antibiotics were unsuccessful in clearing up the infection. Dad had been in the hospital for over eleven weeks. I was so glad he did not know about my diagnosis of multiple sclerosis. He had enough to deal with.

The warmth of the sun soothed my worries as the girls ran about in the park, screaming and laughing as jets of water sprayed them. Our bodies turned golden brown as the summer days rolled by.

"Do you want to go and watch the fireworks again tonight, Rachel?" We discovered by driving a few miles to the north of where we were staying that we gained enough elevation to get a good view of most of the display. It was called "Symphony of Fire" and ran for several weeks. Several countries had taken turns designing the display based out of English Bay on the southwest side of the city. At dusk, two nights a week for several weeks, the skies lit up in a glory of colour and light. To our city-starved eyes, it was spectacular.

"That would be great, Mom. Can we stop and get slushies again? Maybe Becky will be awake this time." This schedule suited Rachel.

Becky was awake at 10.45 pm so we sat on the grass together. Small groups of people gathered in clusters and vehicles parked facing south to see the lights. Some people brought lawn chairs or blankets.

My eyes travelled down the mountain to the water and followed lights from the Lions Gate Bridge, which connected the North and West Shores to Stanley Park, downtown and English Bay. The city was aglow, lit up like a magical Christmas display, city squalor and danger hidden in darkness. The flickering lights of the Seabus, a giant floating "bus" that transported commuters from the downtown core to North Vancouver, was making an evening run across the

82

water. Several miles to the east, a second bridge, aptly named the Second Narrows, spanned the second narrowing of Burrard Inlet and with three lanes in each direction, it eased large volumes of traffic. Vehicle lights wavered in their fleeting passage and the houses nestled in the hills twinkled like stars.

"Pop, bang, pshhhhh." The show had begun. Vivid, colourful arrangements of lights filled the sky as the crowds clapped and cheered. One after another, glowing embers of sparkle trailed the sky after each spectacular rocket ship of light bedazzled its audience. Suddenly it stopped. People began to whisper and talk quietly.

"Is it all done, Mom?" Becky asked as she pulled on my arm. It was hard to tell because each burst of light was glorious and could easily be the finale.

"I'm cold," Rachel said as a new set of fireworks began. I hugged her as we watched the end of the show and then hurried to the car.

It was nearing the end of July and I knew we needed to return home to Robb. I hated to leave without Dad showing any signs of improvement, but we had been gone almost a month. Each day on our trip to the hospital, we drove by the Pacific National Exhibition with its gigantic roller coaster and fairgrounds and I had promised the girls a day on the rides. It was not my idea of fun. Most of the rides made me lightheaded and wobbly, but I knew the girls could ride together while I looked on.

"I'll come on the Ferris-wheel with you. It has a good view of the city," I announced. Rachel was satisfied with my promise.

"Will they have cotton candy?"

"Yes, I think so. I bet we can even get candy apples and those yummy little bite-sized donuts they make while you wait." I could smell the cinnamon already.

The crowd was small and the weather perfect - not too hot - with a gentle ocean breeze. The girls tried a variety of rides and took a break.

"Mom, Mom, you should have heard Rachel scream on the zipper. I didn't like it. I like the swings," Becky said as she looked up at the large swings hanging from long chains that spun around at a moderate speed. "Maybe you could try it with me!" I decided to take a chance, and the three of us grinned at each other as the attendant buckled us in. The operator pulled down a lever. We were raised up into the air slowly and began to spin round. It picked up speed and I gripped the chains.

"Wheeeee," Becky exclaimed as her older sister shouted happily.

"It's fun, hey, Mom? Better than the Ferris-wheel." The backdrop of sparkling ocean, mountains, bridges and homes captivated my attention. The cooling air whipped at the girls' hair and their smiles and whoops of pleasure completed the picture. It was idyllic.

We had had a great visit with my Dad the day before. He was awake, responsive and cheerful. Given all the paraphernalia attached to him, it was so encouraging to see he still had a spark left. Maybe he would recover after all.

I phoned Dave. "We'll be home early next week. My Dad had a good day yesterday. The girls are looking forward to seeing you but not to the long drive. I'll call you before we leave."

Friday was very hot, hotter than I ever remembered the coast to be. I awoke groggy from sleep to hear the phone ringing. It was midnight. Mike's voice sounded far away.

"Kathy, can you come to the hospital right now?

Dad's had a stroke and they don't think he's going to make it through the night. You can bring the kids here." My eyes popped open and my heart raced.

I was galvanized into action, banishing my tiredness. There was no time for shock, grief or worry. The girls bundled into the vehicle, uncomplaining, with their blankets and stuffed animals. Night driving in the city was not too bad with all the lights, but we had a fifteen-minute section of construction to get through, which required all my concentration. Mike's wife met me at the door of their house to take the girls and I sped off to the hospital. I suddenly realized Dad's second wife, Pat, was away in the United States with her daughter, having a break from all the stress.

The room was dim. Dad was covered in blankets with monitors beeping and hospital staff coming and going, while Mike stood by looking very tired. There was no sign of the aide.

"Did you work today?" Mike's job involved shift work and weekends. I had lost track of his schedule.

"Yeah, I'd only been home an hour when the hospital called. I got hold of Paul and I think a buddy's bringing him here."

"You know, I was in on Wednesday and Dad was doing great compared to most days. So this is a shock." I leaned over and rested the back of my hand lightly on Dad's warm forehead.

"Well, all the times I've stopped in recently he's been pretty much out of it."

Paul arrived, looking exhausted after a week of work. I offered to sit with Dad for the first few hours while my brothers slept in the "family" room. They told me that if anything changed with Dad I should come and get them. I prayed that Dad would not just slip away while I sat beside him by myself.

Eventually my head nodded forward and I dozed, only to be woken by two hospital staff as they rolled Dad on one side and then the other to massage his slack muscles. I turned my head away as they efficiently changed his diaper and treated the bedsores on his immune-weakened body. His temperature was up and all the heavy blankets were removed.

The rest of the night was a blur. My brothers kept commenting on how Dad's breathing was becoming shallower, which I barely acknowledged. The three of us reminisced about past adventures together, laughing and joking about the crazy things we did, with Dad's part the highlight – our hero who not only shared life with us but also provided us with experiences that bonded us forever together as family.

"I need to go move my car so it doesn't get towed." I had to get out of the room. Dad had hung on much longer than anyone expected, but I refused to accept that he could die. My mind was hazy.

"Well, okay, Kathy, but don't take too long."

After eating like a robot and using the bathroom, I headed outside into warm sunshine. The heat was already building. Dazed, I found my vehicle ticket-less and drove out of the "night-time only" parking area keeping watch for a daylight-zoned parking spot. I drove around the large park area several times hoping to catch someone leaving, but not one stall became available. I did not have coins for a meter, did not want to risk being towed, and drove about blindly in unfamiliar territory. Desperate, I parked in a tow away zone, when a vehicle pulled out across the street where parking was permitted. I drove two blocks, turned around and secured the spot. The world was spinning and I was fading.

I hurried back into the large hospital and found my

way to Dad's room. The door was wide open and Mike stood at the end of the bed, head hanging.

"He's gone. You took a long time."

"No, no, no" I cried, and ran to my Dad. His pale form was motionless and skin cool to touch. "I'm sorry." Tears ran down my face. Mike's voice broke.

"I'm going home. Paul left five minutes ago."

I could not leave the room so I sat beside my father's body for fifteen minutes. In a trance, I collected a few personal items to take with me, including the red clipboard. The nurse gave me a disinfecting cloth to wipe down the items I took. The "super bug" continued to haunt us in life as well as death. There were further repercussions.

SIX

"The Courage to Change"
~ Al-Anon Family Groups ~

*T*he pain was intense at first. I knew, in my heart, it was the best thing for our father who had suffered so much during the last few years of his life and could now rest peacefully in a better place. It was our turn to suffer the loss of someone who had always been there for us. He had sacrificed himself, nurtured, encouraged and loved us unconditionally. He was a man who had loved life and made the best of each situation, found good qualities in people before he saw their flaws, and genuinely cared for people. Perhaps at times he was too nice and kind, and even an "enabler" in some relationships, but his positive outlook helped him to cope with life's trials.

I phoned Dave with the news. "Dad passed away this morning. He had a stroke last night. " My voice was numb with grief.

"I'm sorry, Kathy." Dave sounded sincere. He knew how highly I regarded my father.

"I guess we'll be delayed a few more days. We don't have a date set for the funeral yet. We're waiting for Pat to arrive, so I'll let you know when I find out. I can hardly wait to get home."

The day of the service was beautiful, as were the flowers and small chapel in West Vancouver. Mike, Paul and I had put together a collage of pictures representing some of the highlights of Dad's life, and it was set up on an easel in the foyer. Because of the circumstances, Dad was to be cremated, but for some reason I felt he should be with us during the service and the rental of a coffin had been arranged. We arrived early. Fragrant, light perfume filled the air.

I surveyed the lovely display of flowers at the front of the chapel with satisfaction, remembering how much Dad treasured flowers, shrubs and gardens.

"Where is the coffin?" I asked. The director of the chapel led me off to the side behind a curtain.

"Here" he said, motioning with his hand.

I stared with disbelief at the ugly Styrofoam box resting on a stand with wheels.

"What is this? We were supposed to have a traditional wooden coffin." The director said he would find out and disappeared.

A few minutes later, another man arrived with the funeral director to explain the situation.

"Because of the MRSA, we were unable to put your father's body in a rented coffin. It's considered contaminated, and must be disposed of along with whatever receptacle the body is placed in." Not only did the super bug strip our father of dignity while he was alive but also in death. I understood the living needed to be protected from potential health risks, but could we not have been informed in advance? This was such an important day. My hands shook and there was a bitter taste in my mouth.

The funeral service to honour my father's life was moments away from beginning so I pushed my frustration aside. My brothers did the same. Michael had done a wonderful job of preparing a keepsake pamphlet with a picture of "Len" smiling on the cover, a poem inside that I had written, and a beautiful verse on the back that Mike had composed. Dad's body lay hidden from view as we listened to the minister and shared in this important grieving ceremony with family and friends. After a light luncheon and exchange of condolences, my daughters and I quickly changed for the trip home to Alberta. My mother-in-law had slipped out quietly after the service. I was so grateful she had given us her home to stay in while she was away because it had been a refuge for us.

~~~~~~

The heat was intense as we travelled north through the interior of BC and gained latitude. My goal was to get to Clearwater, north of Kamloops, and we drove almost until dark. Floods of tears kept washing over me and my kids let me cry. I could not believe the timing of my father's death. If he had hung on another week we would have gone back to Alberta, and I would have had to make the long journey again. It had been another blessing.

At home, there was plenty of work to be done and I threw myself into busy-ness. It was an elixir for me, a way to cope and work through grieving. I was beginning to think more about my diagnosis of multiple sclerosis, and knew it was time to resign from the fire department, given my inconsistent energy levels and lack of confidence in my physical ability. Even though I still felt strong most of the time, the stress involved in some of the calls would affect me. At least I knew why my balance was off. I had to hold onto the wall to put on my firefighting gear. The stiffness was obvious to me as I crawled around on top of the fire truck to help relay hose. I shared my news with a few of the members.

"There's a lot you can still do. We need people here at the base on almost every emergency, manning the radios," the captain said.

"I don't know. I need to think about it some more." My stint as a radio operator working for Forestry in past summers had given me a good feel for the job and the excitement was almost addictive, but I was unsure about the commitment at this point in my life. The job would be highly disruptive, creating more stress than I could handle.

Life on the Coal Branch carried on as it always had. The weather was hot and Dave was encouraged by steady tipi and boat rentals. It was not enough to generate a profit but definitely a step in the right direction.

On my way to Edson one day, I passed the Coal Branch Cemetery, and fresh tears for my loss poured down my cheeks, the first in many days. I was surprised how quickly my tears had lessened after the initial emotions of losing Dad had subsided, but I had grieved intensely at the beginning until there was nothing left to feel. At least the rawness had eased. The recent construction of the local cemetery reminded me of the many funerals I had attended over the past five years, which in a way had helped prepare me for my own loss.

Before I knew it, September had arrived and Rachel was riding the school bus to Edson early each morning.

"So, what do you think, Rachel?" I asked after her first week.

"It's great, it's cool, way better than the Bryan School, and I've made some new friends. I've been invited to a sleepover at Jessica's house and I really want to go. Can I please, Mom?" Rachel went home with her new friend after school the following Friday and I picked up a very tired, happy kid on Saturday. Becky and I had done some shopping in Edson first.

The busy season for camping was over. I had worked

hard at bringing the accounting up to date. Dave and I did not discuss the fact that another season had passed and we were still in the red, despite good sales. More changes loomed for tenure of the land and I left it for Dave to determine what needed to be done.

My part-time teacher assistant job began in early September, the day after Becky's fourth birthday. It was great to be back. Steven had turned ten years old. He was much bigger and heavier than the little boy I had started out with so his mother, the teachers and I worked on some strategies for managing transfers from vehicle, wheelchair, floor and desk. I was grateful for the wheelchair ramp that had been built to accommodate special-needs kids, and thought about the stairs his mother had to negotiate each day to move her son from home to vehicle. The family was looking into various means to manage their son's growing size and weight. I could see many challenges ahead.

The school closure was looming. Parents formed a group to continue fighting the decision, but there were few people involved. Currently, I was a part-time employee with no children of my own attending, and I had mixed feelings about the future of a school with only fifteen students. Were we doing our kids a disservice by offering them a shrinking school with shrinking programming? How much could we cut and still meet the curriculum? What about the projections for a continuing drop in student numbers? Yet how could we let our young children ride the bus two hours a day to school on the heavy industrial-use highway? Either way, there were sacrifices to be made. It was part of rural living.

One of the teachers and I seemed to have a lot in common when it came to the men in our lives, and we had had several insightful discussions after passing comments back and forth that made me realize how many unhappy marriages there were. Sally had recently split with her husband. She had had been married before and had grown children.

"But how did you decide it was time to split up?" Sally frowned and shook her head.

"I'd had enough of the crazy behaviour, moodiness, anger and depression. It reached a point where I'd run out of ways to deal with all the problems and I felt like I was no longer 'me,' consumed by another person's needs, wants and desires." This sounded so familiar it was frightening.

"Did you consider how you were going to pay the bills on only one income?"

"It helped that my parents left me some money when they passed away. I think that empowered me to make the decision." I thought about the money I had put away from my mother's estate, even though some was gone on the purchase of a four-wheel drive vehicle. Ever since my accident, a four-by-four was something on my "much desired list" and the inheritance had made this dream possible. It was a luxury many considered a necessity on the back roads.

"Even with the money I've put away, I couldn't possibly support myself and two kids on a part-time salary." Sally smiled.

"That's true. You'd have to work full-time." We took advantage of the rare empty classroom and shared more about our lives. My diagnosis of MS came up but I brushed it aside as a minor concern. So far, I had only been forced to give up skating and long-distance walking, which had very little effect on my outlook.

There was coolness in the air and frost on the ground in the mornings. The leaves on the trees began turning shades of yellow and orange. Huckleberries were in abundance. We reaped the benefits of Dave's love of growing vegetables in a wonderful harvest of carrots and greenhouse tomatoes, and the fall quest for firewood was lessened by excess brought in from the campground. It was dark when Rachel got up at 6.30 am, and soon the evening light would decrease as winter solstice crept in. At first, it was subtle, but by November, a dramatic loss of daylight hours signalled the onset of winter.

Towards the end of September, I walked into the tiny office of the Bryan School, awaiting the arrival of Steven. Sally handed me a fax.

"There's a teacher assistant job for you in Edson," she joked. I read the posting and gave her a puzzled look.

"But it's full-time. I only work part-time," I said doubtfully.

"Kathy, you could easily transfer within the school division if you wanted to, part-time or full-time, you know. That would be within Edson, Hinton, Jasper and Grande Cache. This time of year, postings come up steady for teaching assistants. I'll save the faxes that come in, if you like." My head was spinning with the implications.

For the rest of the week, Sally handed me posting after posting, jobs varying in nature, some specialized and tied to one student, others general classroom aides with a variety of duties. Most were at the elementary level. I had doubts, but also felt confident and recognized that I was capable. I'd always thought Jasper would be an awesome place to live with its stunning Rocky Mountain scenery and interesting mix of people.

"Here's one for you. It's in Hinton at a school where Stephen is currently the principal. That would work, Kathy!" Stephen had been a teacher and the principal of the Bryan School when Rachel was in grades three, four and five, and I knew him personally. He was also Sally's ex-husband. His creative disciplinary style, high energy and confidence inspired the students. I had enjoyed his time with us. Parents and students alike either loved him, or did not like him at all, and Rachel, Dave and I liked him immediately. Rachel had done well under his care and guidance.

But Hinton? It was an industrial pulp-mill town, surrounded by coalmines, set in the foothills of the Rockies. It was an attractive town despite the mill, and had many services that we had lived without for almost ten years, such as a hospital, mall, restaurants and a wonderful recreation center with a pool and skating rink.

"Would I apply to Stephen, directly?" I asked.

"Yes, you need a resume and cover letter. We could send it from here. I'm not sure why I'm telling you all this, Kathy. We don't want to lose you, you know."

"Well, I have to think about it, anyway. Thanks," I said as I stuffed the piece of paper into my backpack.

On Friday afternoon, I stood in the office holding my resume tightly. This could change my future. Was it the right thing to do? I nervously eyed the "send" key on the fax machine. Sally had run off to help a student, so I stood alone questioning my actions. Suddenly, I hit the send key and breathed a sigh of relief - no more second-guessing or over-analyzing things. In my heart, I was excited and as sure as I could be that this was what I should do.

Monday was the earliest I anticipated hearing any news as I calmly went about my tasks and basked in the warm fall sunshine. At dinnertime on Saturday, I was barbequing on the back deck when Rachel poked her head out the door and handed me the phone.

"For you, Mom." Rachel disappeared into the yard.

"Hello."

"Hi, Kathy. This is Stephen Angle. How are you?" My heart started beating faster.

"Hi Stephen. I'm pretty good. Did you get my fax?"

"I did, and the job's yours, if you want it." I gasped in surprise.

"You mean, I don't need an interview, just like that? You're going to hire me?" He laughed.

"Yep, it's that easy. Let me know when you decide, and we'll work out the details."

It was an opportunity to get out of a destructive marriage and a shrinking community that offered less and less to families as schools and industry closed their doors permanently. This alone outweighed all the risks and unknowns the future might hold. I was fearful of my family's reaction and especially Dave's. I knew Dawn and Steven's family would be disappointed, but in nine months, my job at the Bryan School would be ending unless I was willing to travel to Edson and back each day. By Monday, I knew with certainty what action I should take. I accepted the job.

I felt as though I had stepped over the edge of a cliff. I was freefalling into uncharted territory like a bird that has not yet learned to fly, madly flapping its wings in an attempt to stay airborne, with no guarantee of a soft landing. I thought after having made the right decision some peace might come my way, but instead my brain switched to fast-forward with doubt after doubt taunting me until exhaustion finally took over and I succumbed to the healing power of sleep. Dave would be devastated and I did not know how or when to tell him. What would Rachel choose? I would not force her to come with me.

The following weekend, the dreaded moment finally came. Dave sat staring blankly at me while Rachel broke into loud violent sobs and ran out the front door.

"I knew something was up, but you're *leaving??* Where will you go?" Dave's voice rose. The unreal scene continued.

"I've accepted a full-time teacher assistant job at a school in Hinton, starting next week. It's considered a transfer from Robb, within the school division." Silence. The wall clock ticked loudly in my ears.

"Are you taking the girls?"

"That's Rachel's decision, but since the school's closing here, it makes sense that they come with me." My voice shook and I was racked with guilt. I was destroying a family but I felt as though I had been destroyed too by the insanity of violence, lies, and opposite views of the world. Who would have guessed it would turn out like this? I had been so sure I could help this troubled man see a better vision, but at what cost to myself?

Rachel's reaction scared me. Maybe she would want to stay in Robb and continue taking the bus to Edson. She really liked her new school. A neighbour phoned.

"Rachel's here. She's very upset. When she's ready, maybe you could come and get her or Tina could bring her over." I appreciated her concern for my daughter, and lack of questions.

"Thanks, Anita. Would you let me know when she's ready to come home?"

Dave disappeared into the detached barn-style garage that sat behind the house. It had been our first building project. I looked around at the beautiful home we had built together and wished things had turned out differently. We had both tried everything we knew to make it work, but unhappiness prevailed and filtered down to the kids, making it even harder.

I expected far more opposition and anger from Dave,

but his resigned detachedness allowed me to proceed. He slept on the couch that night and every night after until we left a month later. Rachel adjusted to the plan very quickly. She had secretly wanted to leave the small town for a long time. There was so little for kids her age to do. Some families travelled back and forth to town for their children's activities, but I doubted we would be doing a lot of that given Dave's attitude about limiting trips to town, my dislike of winter driving, and our restricted budget.

Was I sad to be leaving? I had spent one quarter of my life in this small tightly knit community and had made some wonderful friends. I felt guilty for wanting to go, but realized it was the people I would miss, not the lifestyle and isolation. So no, I was not sad. In fact, I wanted to celebrate.

Leaving Robb solved my dilemma about the fire department, and I attended my last meeting before the big moving day. I was presented with a wall plaque. *"In appreciation of your commitment, dedication and unending support for 10 years to the Robb Volunteer Fire Department."* The names of the members were engraved into the shiny, blue metal plate mounted on a wooden firefighter crest. It meant a lot.

The girls and I were very excited about living in a place with "amenities" and basic services most people took for granted. I arranged to stay with friends for three weeks while Rachel and I adjusted to a new school, and we found a place to live. Becky stayed with her Dad, while Rachel and I returned on Friday afternoons to spend weekends in Robb, getting organized to move and taking small loads of things back with us to Hinton. Dave did not try to stop me and even helped load a few things into the pickup truck. I was no longer afraid. The biggest challenge was finding a place to live.

We started looking at apartment rentals but did not find anything that felt "just right." One of the landlords suggested checking with a realtor, who directed us to a few house-rental options. We looked at a tiny house across from the high school where Rachel would attend and only three blocks from the school where I worked.

"Have you considered buying a house?" the realtor asked. "Sometimes you can purchase with only five percent down, and the mortgage wouldn't be much more than a monthly rental." It was a good question.

"I hadn't thought of that possibility. I do have a bit of money saved that I guess I could use for a down payment. That certainly increases the options."

We figured out the price range I could afford and arranged to view what was available. Rachel came with me. The third and last option we looked at was just right for us. It was an older, single story three-bedroom home in a beautiful neighbourhood, close to both schools. It had a huge yard, lots of trees, sidewalks and the Recreation Center only two blocks away.

In less than three weeks, we moved in. We hardly had any furniture, and the girls slept on pieces of foam on the floor. It did not matter; we were safe, warm and had a kitchen table to eat our meals at. There was a daycare at the Recreation Center where I was able to take Becky each day before work, and I applied for a government subsidy, knowing I would be unable to pay the full cost. I was worried we would not be able to afford this new life so I counted every penny.

In the meantime, we owned the house. It seemed unreal. I mentally thanked my mom for the small inheritance she left me – it had been one of the keys to unlocking the door of change and new direction.

The weeks flew by. I liked my new job and was

becoming more familiar with the role an assistant played in the classroom as I scurried from the upper floor of grade four and five, to the opposite end of lower elementary, where the grade one classroom where I spent an hour each day was located. The kids were full of energy, curious and funny. Some were quiet and soft spoken while others could not sit still or remain quiet for long. I held a student's hand as we walked down the hall to the washroom.

"Will it be recess soon?" she asked. I glanced at my watch.

"Only fifteen more minutes. Be quick and you'll have time to finish your work." I stood outside the bathroom and looked out of the window at the swirling snow. It was not my turn to go outside for supervision today, so I could relax a little when the bell rang and I headed down to the staff-room for a quick coffee. I did not know fifteen minutes could disappear so fast.

I thought back to my first day and how overwhelming it had been. The school had almost four hundred students, forty staff, a gymnasium, music room, library, computer labs and twenty classrooms. It was a huge change from the two-room school I had started out in. The principal took me on a grand tour and we ended up back in his office. Stephen asked me about multiple sclerosis. He had heard.

"I was diagnosed in June. But I still feel very strong and am managing just fine so far," I said a little defensively. I had not had much time to think about it.

"I'm sure you'll do well. We're looking forward to having you on staff." I appreciated his confidence in me, and his upfront approach. The diagnosis was not something I was comfortable with yet. It was too new. I knew I could count on Steve to be discreet.

There was an Al-Anon group very close to our house

and I began attending the weekly meetings to continue growing and healing, making new friends and sharing in fellowship via common ground. We started each meeting with the Lord's Prayer and followed through by working on the 12-Steps and applying them to our own circumstances. Personal stories would often move me to tears and I was grateful for a higher power and the encouragement that slogans offered. "Just for today I will try to live through this day only, and not try and tackle all my problems at once." Look where faith, trust and courage had led us.

SEVEN

"Remind me each day that the race is not
always to the swift, that there is more to life
than increasing its speed."
~ Orin L. Crain ~

*B*y the time Christmas came, I was ready for the two-week break. Separation made the celebration awkward. The girls wanted to stay in their new house, so I invited Dave to stay overnight on Christmas Eve. With the dwindling inheritance money, I bought a cheap futon to put in the living room that served as a sleeping place for guests. A couple of chairs and a small side table hardly filled the large room. The ancient furnace was noisy, the windows were single-paned and draughty, and the add-on kitchen was freezing compared to the rest of the house. We turned up the heat but it was still freezing. The bathroom had been modernized, the walls were freshly painted and it was clean. I planned to upgrade slowly.

When the girls went back to Robb with their Dad for a few days, I took the opportunity to get organized, and I slept in and read. The local library had several books on multiple sclerosis and I picked one called "Running the Distance," written by a young woman diagnosed in her twenties. I was thirty-nine and learned the average age of diagnosis was between twenty and forty.

The story was insightful, moving and inspiring even though I did not relate personally to the circumstances. The author was younger, single and eventually developed a pronounced limp upon walking any distance. Even though my legs felt heavy after walking several kilometres, I did not have a limp or any other disability that anyone noticed. The word *progressive* in the context of the disease had little meaning to me.

Feeling particularly strong one day and determined to outwit my body, I coaxed Becky into an outing at the local indoor skating rink. I still owned figure skates and we borrowed a pair for Becky to wear. Carefully, we stepped onto the rink, staying close to the sideboards and clear of other skaters.

"Mom, my feet hurt," Becky cried, as I gauged my balance and pushed off. It was not bad, but I went very slowly. Becky took my hand and we moved forward until she lost her balance and went down onto the ice. The padded snowsuit cushioned her fall. A young child skated by us and held tightly to a metal-framed walker. It reminded me of the wooden chair with metal legs Rachel used to push around when she was learning to skate.

"Hey, Beck, look at that. Would you like to try it?" She hesitated. "I'll see if there's one we can use. Stay right here."

I returned with the funny-looking contraption and we spent a few minutes trying it out. When Becky was comfortable, I ventured off on my own to skate to the other end of the rink, shaky but determined to recapture my past love of skating. Becky fell several times and pushed the walker away in disgust. I helped her to the bench.

"I didn't like that walker, Mom. It made me fall. Can I just sit here for a while?" This was not going as well as I had hoped, but I took advantage of the moment and set out again, glancing back at Becky as I skated. She was chewing on a finger of her glove. "Wham, crash." A young skater clipped my right skate with her walker and I went down hard, falling on my hip and hitting my forehead. It scared me and I realized the walkers were dangerous. They were a contradiction of hindrance and help. It was not a good place for slow, unsteady legs.

Disillusioned, we left. Both my body and ego were bruised and I retired my skates with only a little regret. It was time to be realistic. My stubbornness would defeat me if I were not careful.

We tried cross-country skiing at the local golf course, but the cold sank into my bones and Becky certainly did not like it. I waited for a weekend with milder temperatures and soft snow when Becky was with her Dad and set out on my own, determined to make use of my skis and get some fresh air and exercise. The familiar pattern returned. I made a good strong start, had a tiring middle and felt exhaustion at the end. I tumbled into the soft, cold snow, became chilled and started a vicious cycle of falls, frustration and reduced stamina that served to discourage me even more. Over the course of the winter, I attempted several more expeditions. Instead of building up my strength as I had hoped, I became weaker each time. I retired my cross-country skis to the shed.

For the whole of my life, being active had given me confidence, kept me in shape and helped me release anger and frustration. I was drawn to solitary sports where I did not have to depend on others and could set my own pace and expectations. Even though team sports were sometimes fun, my preference was to go solo. So not only was MS challenging a lifestyle I was passionate about but it went against social expectation that being fit was the ideal for everyone. How could I change a lifetime of internal and external conditioning? Every time I tried to build up strength doing an activity I liked, even something as simple as walking, it felt as though my body turned against me as fatigue set in. Recently, a "pins and needles" sensation had invaded the inside of my legs, invisible to all, but distracting my brain and my feet were always freezing and even numb. The strange prickling was pronounced at night, after I exercised and stopped to rest.

After Christmas, the vice-principal asked me to come to her office.

"So what do you think of our busy school, Kathy?"

"It's great. I know my way around pretty good now." I wondered what she wanted to talk to me about. She read my mind.

"I have a proposal for you. I understand you've expressed interest in working with our special needs student Melissa, who is in grade two, and we actually need someone to work half a day with her starting right away. What do you think?"

"What would be involved in her care?" I had seen Melissa in the hallways and liked her pretty smile. Her walk was off, kind of a lunge-lurch affair, but she was quick and remained upright when I had seen her.

"She needs full supervision during recess and lunch hour, as well as classroom time. You would be job sharing with another aide, who works with Melissa in the morning. The focus is on toilet training. Your duties would include taking her to gym, music and computers with the rest of the class. She also participates in community programming, which at this time involves taking Melissa to the local pool." I was comfortable in the pool environment, so this was not a problem.

"Is she on medication?"

"Yes, she takes that at home, for seizures."

"Oh. How often does she have seizures?"

"Very infrequently. I think she's had two since school started." It sounded like Melissa was much more medically stable than the first child I had worked with in Robb.

"Does she feed herself?"

"Yes. She needs a bit of help opening things, and some coaxing sometimes."

"And where's Melissa at verbally?" I had already decided I wanted to do it.

'She has some language, uses a few words and we are working on developing her communication. We're not always sure what she understands."

I was tired of moving from classroom to classroom throughout the day, from one end of the school to the other, so not only would this be closer to what I wanted to do - working with special needs kids - it would save all that running back and forth.

"Yes. I'll do it."

"Thanks, Kathy. You can start on Monday. Melissa's aide, Shirley, and her grade two teacher will help you get familiarized."

This newest job development motivated me to get to the pool that very weekend. Rachel did not want to join us, so Becky and I went during "family swim" and spent some time together splashing in the kiddie pool. There was one lane set up for length swimming in the big pool and very few swimmers. I wondered if it would wear me out because it had been years since I had done any distance swimming. The lifeguard agreed to watch Becky for a short time while I tried it. I did six sidestrokes and six breaststrokes. It felt great. I added laps until I found my comfort zone. I had finally found something I could do that did not exhaust me!

We stopped in the library where I took the opportunity to research some information on Melissa's condition. She was born with microcephaly. I did not know what to expect.

"Microcephaly is a medical condition in which the circumference of the head is smaller than normal because the brain has not developed properly or has stopped growing. Depending on the severity of the accompanying syndrome, children with microcephaly may have mental retardation, delayed motor functions and speech, facial distortions, short stature, hyperactivity, seizures, difficulties with coordination and balance and other neurological abnormalities."

Melissa did not have all those problems but she definitely had speech and motor delays that would present some big challenges. The National Institute of Neurological Disorders and Stroke (NINDS) information page noted:

"Early childhood intervention programs that involve physical, speech and occupational therapists help maximize abilities and minimize dysfunction. Medications are often used to control seizures."

I knew Melissa was on medication but was unsure what other specialists were involved in her support.

Melissa did not like me at first because I was a stranger thrown into her world without any warning. I was disappointed but guessed that with a little time, things would improve. She was quiet and withdrawn when I was around, although she responded well to verbal cues and routine.

The adults familiar with Melissa described her basic needs and capabilities. Just like working with Steven at the Bryan School, the day-to-day individual programming was wide open to ideas. Once again, it was adapt, modify and adjust to the child's individual needs while attempting to include the child in as many activities as possible in the classroom. As I was to learn, the inclusion of all children within their age group was fraught with challenges that only seemed to intensify as they grew older and the gaps grew bigger.

In February, I turned forty, a milestone birthday. Dave invited me out to dinner and I accepted his conciliatory gesture, hoping I was not giving the wrong impression. The separation was still fresh, like a breath of fresh air for me, and I finally felt freed from chains of fear and worry that had bound me constantly in our marriage. I was never good enough - not strong, fast, or smart enough for Dave.

Becky spent weekends with her Dad once or twice a month, but I could not convince Rachel to go back on any regular basis.

"I hate it there, Mom. There's nothing to do, and my only close friend is busy with her own stuff and never around." Tina was a few years older and in high school with a different group of friends.

"I thought you might hang out with Dad and Becky, but I guess that's pretty boring. Maybe you could go if there's something interesting happening." Sometimes the community organized events during special holidays that often included kids. Dave had expressed his disappointment at Rachel's lack of interest in spending any time with him, but since the same thing was happening at our house, it was her age more than anything that was causing the changes. Friends became the first priority, parents were not cool and even little sisters were a pain. I was too busy juggling my responsibilities to dwell on this for long. Teenagers go through many changes, as I was to learn.

The children in Melissa's grade two class were performing a song at a local senior's home, which the kids walked to after lunch.

"How far do you think it is, Shirley?" I asked my co-worker.

"Not very far, Kathy. I don't think we'll have any problem. It's not cold, and Melissa's family brought in her three-wheeled, all-terrain jogger that we could take turns pushing. Hopefully the sidewalks will be shovelled." It had snowed the night before.

"I hope you're right. It might be a bit tricky in places." It was clear and crisp outside, about minus ten degrees Celsius, I estimated, and the sun shone brilliantly. I walked in the middle of the group led by the teacher, while Shirley and Melissa followed in the jogger as the kids chatted to each other. By the time the lodge was in sight, my feet were frozen and a cold wind had begun to swirl the snow around. I heard Melissa laughing and I turned around and smiled. Two of the students were pushing her as Shirley walked close by. Soon we were in the warm lodge and it felt good to sit down.

On the return trip, it was my turn to supervise Melissa. I discovered pushing the jogger made walking somehow easier. Some of the students asked to take a turn pushing and I unwillingly turned over the handle. Before we could see the school, my feet were numb and dragging. I took over the jogger and dropped slightly behind the group, alarmed at my tired legs and the exhaustion that had overtaken my body. In a blur, we got inside the school.

"You go for your break now, Kathy, and I'll watch Melissa," her teacher suggested.

"Thanks, Pat." I was grateful for the chance to rest and ducked into the small kitchen down the hall, where no one was working. I closed the door, grateful to be alone. I pulled an orange out of my bag and sat gazing out of the window. My toes were warming up and my left leg was tingling, but the weakness in my legs scared me. Thank goodness the workday was almost over.

~~~~~~

One day unexpectedly my brother Paul called from Vancouver. We had gone our separate ways as adults and had only seen each other at infrequent family gatherings, so his call took me by surprise.

"Hey Kath, how's it going? Do you like your new place? I can't believe you really made the move." He paused for my reply.

"You know what, Paul, we love it here. So things are going well and this little house is ideal for us. It's really close to everything - work, schools, stores and the Recreation Center. It's a beautiful old neighbourhood surrounded by churches and trees. The only drawback is the pulp mill that's close by, but it's part of what drives the community and besides, what place is perfect? Fortunately, we don't smell it very often."

"I know, for me it's these crazy car alarms and the train. It's way too noisy here, and even though I love the area, I need to move. I hate moving."

We talked about our lives and the irony of both being on our own. Paul was twice divorced and had no children. Health issues were surfacing compounded by his past problems with alcohol and drug addiction. I thought about the Narcotics Anonymous meeting I had attended with him after he learned of my experience with a 12-Step Program (Al-Anon) that had helped me out of the trenches. A survivor, I had been honoured to attend, as this was a rare trust my brother had placed in me.

Paul asked me several times how I was feeling and I

110

knew my diagnosis of MS bothered him.

"I feel good. I can do almost everything I used to and I have started swimming lengths at the pool. Of course I'm tired when things get hectic, but anyone would be tired." I left out the details about numbness and tingling.

"Yeah, I'm not feeling great these days myself. I work way too much and need to focus more on my health. I did buy a mountain bike, though, and that should help me get into shape. I work out at the gym a lot, too. There are some stupid tests I had to go for at the hospital but I haven't heard anything back." It was another thing we had in common - health concerns. I sometimes wondered how Paul's body could stand up to the substance abuse inflicted upon it. The few times he had opened up and shared bits and pieces of his past made me shudder in horror. It made my partying days seem harmless. I prayed he had a grip on his demons. Even though he professed to be in control, his actions showed otherwise. Powerless, remember, Paul? Work the program.

Reconnecting with Paul was wonderful. We reminisced about the past, laughed over some of the adventures we had shared, and gained a new respect for one another. It was almost like talking to an old friend. We had things in common again that might go a long way towards bridging the gap that had grown over the years.

~~~~~~

The school year ended in June. I was pleased with the relationship Melissa and I had established. She accepted, trusted and depended on me and I looked forward to seeing her each day. Becky would start kindergarten in the fall at the school where I worked. Rachel was moving on to high school.

Time off from the regular busy routine was reviving. We had lots of family and friends visit, and the weather was lovely. I bought a lawn mower and took great pride in keeping the grass cut. I added a small flowerbed and a few shrubs. The back yard was huge, with a couple of big old trees and a fire pit. Six scraggly old spruce trees shaded the front yard, and I dug a triangle-shaped garden in a corner beneath my bedroom window. It was relaxing and satisfying to watch the gardens come to life.

Kelly-Leigh came for a visit from Ontario and brought her dog, Copper, a beautiful Cocker Spaniel with soulful brown eyes. We spent an evening laughing, sharing stories and reminiscing about the past. Out came the yearbooks and the shoebox full of keepsakes I had stored away and kept for almost thirty years. Rachel and Becky found it highly entertaining.

"Let's do some local exploring, Kathy. What's close by that might be interesting?"

"You might like Switzer Provincial Park, about a twenty-minute drive west and then north. There are some beautiful lakes, trails and stunning scenery."

After enjoying our time at the Park, the following day we travelled together to the city of Edmonton, and went to an annual festival called Klondike Days. Smells of grilled burgers, hotdogs, and popcorn drifted through the gates of the amusement park, and we decided to do the "log-run" to cool off in the heat of the day. Four of us packed into a carved-out log, and we prepared to get wet. Screaming and laughing as the ride propelled us down a steep channel, we continued to build on our history of adventure together, now adding my daughters to the fun. Of course, no trip to Edmonton could be complete without visiting West Edmonton Mall, famous for its massive size, the indoor water park, wave pool and water slides, mini-golf, skating rink, amusement park, deep sea adventure park, movie theatre and miles of stores all under one roof. Shopping was the highlight, as Kelly-Leigh took each girl to her favourite store and bought practical, high quality clothing that they picked out. She was their star. It was Auntie Kelly-Leigh from there on in. She spoiled me too.

"You're an amazing friend. My girls just loved your visit. We did so much in four days. Thanks for everything."

"My pleasure, sweetie. Your daughters are lots of fun, smart and special. I had a riot with them. Hope we can do something every year together." Kelly-Leigh hugged and kissed us all before she zoomed off in the rental car with Copper to catch a plane back to Ontario. She had a busy veterinary practice to get back to.

I lay in bed that night thinking about the past and how oddly lives grow apart and become intertwined again and how lucky I was, that, despite MS, my life was so full. I was trying to pinpoint the time when my first symptom had appeared, long before the diagnosis and subtly hidden in the busyness of life. What was it? I thought about the many walks Dave and I had taken in our early adult relationship and his comments about the "funny way I walked." It was hard for me to judge, even though friends and family had never made such an observation. I took it personally, almost like an insult, as my competitive spirit rejected such an idea and my athletic aptitude denied such a possibility. Was there something in his observation? How could I have continued to do all the things I did for a further fifteen years, before I noticed anything askew myself? The list of activities went on and on in my head like hiking in the mountains, walking long distances, biking, swimming, skiing, skating, tennis, badminton, jogging –

I couldn't have had MS then, could I?
~~~~~~

The cold steel ten-step ladder mounted to the wall ran straight up to the second floor cupola. I heard my call sign loudly over the radio.

"XMA286 this is XMA35. How do you copy?" I dropped the knife on the counter and scrambled up the ladder. I knew I should not have come down to make a sandwich. The fire hazard was high and still climbing. On the third rung, my foot slipped and I banged my knee hard. I stopped to realign myself and continued up. I hit my other knee on the top rung. I reached the radio out of breath and called the radio operator.

"XMA35 this is XMA286. Did you call here?" I rubbed my stinging left knee.

"Hi Kathy, we had a smoke reported in southwest of 4922. Could you check that area for us, please?"

Funny, there had been no missed footing on the ladder the summer before. The second summer at the Forestry Lookout, though, I not only missed my footing on the ladder, I actually fell off it when I missed a rung altogether and dropped a foot or so back to the floor. I was not hurt but could not blame it on the slippery metal this time. I let the memory fade and put it on "the back burner" to simmer for a while. If I did not force it, more would come. Insignificant little incidents now had importance. I would return to that idea again at some point in the future to see what else might be buried there.
~~~~~~

My friend Alison arrived to stay for a week, with her twin boys Christopher and Curtis, and we settled in for a time of adventure, good food, wine and conversation. Her boys and my youngest daughter were the same age, and I have a great picture of the three of them standing in the bathroom brushing their teeth together, just tall enough to spit into the sink.

"So, Kathy, did you tell me you still have some of

your stuff in Robb? Do you want to get it?" I thought about it for a minute.

"You know, it's probably my last chance. Most of it is furniture from my mother's estate." It had been almost eight months since I had left and Dave was not happy about the separation. This would be one more thing to anger him. I would risk it.

"I could rent a truck for the day. Would you help me?"

"Sure. Can Rachel look after the kids?"

"That's a great idea. I'll try and make all the arrangements." The details fell into place, and I called Dave to let him know we were coming. He did not sound impressed and planned to be out. I was relieved. Al and I could handle all the stuff, two strong women on a mission!

There was an old walnut dining room suite with a huge buffet, six chairs, a china cabinet, lots of smaller furniture items, and a beautiful area rug. We packed all the stuff into the back of a pickup truck, heaving and straining with the heavy, bulky buffet, but somehow managed to fit everything in and tie it down for the fifty-kilometre ride on a dusty logging road back to Hinton. It was quite a workout unloading everything at the other end into our little house and delivering the rental truck back in time, but we managed. My neighbour probably shook his head when he saw the truck backed up on the front lawn, but our scruffy barren space was no match to his beautiful lawn so a few tire tracks would not change much. Doing it this way, we were almost at the front door and able to slide the heavy, awkward pieces in ourselves. I felt physically strong but mentally drained. It was another move away from the marriage.

Alison and the boys left for Vancouver a few days

later. It was a thousand-kilometre drive and with kids, she planned to take two days. I was surprised to hear Alison's voice a day later when I picked up the phone.

"We had an accident on the highway, a rollover. We're okay, but the car's totalled." Her voice broke. I was shocked.

"You're sure you guys are all right? Where did it happen?" I imagined driving off to help until I found out they were hundreds of kilometres from us. Alison was crying.

"It happened so fast, on a curve when this guy was passing us. I really don't quite know how it could have happened. It's so unreal." She was in shock.

"Have you called anyone in your family?" She had parents, a brother and sister in Vancouver, again hundreds of kilometres from Alison and the twins.

"Yes. But my friend Neil's coming to get us since he can leave right away." I did not know Neil, but I knew he cared about Alison. She had been divorced for a few years. "We're staying in a hotel tonight in Quesnel."

We talked a bit more and then I hung up. Alison was a responsible, careful driver and ironically a claims adjuster for automobile accidents. I thanked God that they were only shaken up. Accidents were horrific events that I had seen from both perspectives - victim and rescuer. Goosebumps covered my arms. Life was scary at times.

Life was also exciting because it was 1999, almost the turn of the century, and the world was busy planning huge celebrations. I decided the girls and I needed to do something special to commemorate the year 2000 so we discussed the idea of a trip.

"What do you think about travelling to Nova Scotia next summer to see David and Helene?" I looked at Rachel expectantly. They had been a big part of her life until moving away to the East Coast when Rachel was eight years old.

"Yes, that might be fun, Mom. What would we do?"

"I'll talk to Helene about the possibilities. What interests you?" Rachel thought for a minute.

"I like shopping, beaches and cool places like Klondike Days."

"Becky, do you want to go on a trip with us next summer? Auntie Kelly-Leigh said she'll be in New Brunswick in July, which is close to Nova Scotia, and maybe we could see her too." Becky nodded her head agreeably. None of us had ever been to the east coast of Canada.

The school year started and we fell into a slightly different routine. Becky went a half-day to kindergarten, and Rachel started high school. After rural living for ten years, the novelty of having amenities so close had not worn off. We were making new friends and settling into our "new beginnings."

EIGHT

"O Canada!
Our Home and Native Land…"
~ Canadian Anthem ~

Becky and I often walked to school in the morning, and I walked three blocks home at lunch for a short break from the hectic school environment. I switched to driving at this point in the day to save on time and energy, picking my daughter up from daycare after school and running errands.

Through luck, fate or God's plan, my good friend Bernadette and her family moved to Hinton in the fall. We had a special connection because we had kids the same age and we both worked in schools. Once they were settled, she called me.

"Hi, Kathy. I was wondering if you, Becky and Rachel would like to come for dinner on Saturday. Then we can visit while the kids play."

"That sounds awesome! We'd love to. How's everything going at your new school?"

"Oh, it's kind of crazy but I've got lots of help so hopefully that will compensate. Teaching grade one is very different from kindergarten and I have tons of prep work to do. It's a huge commitment."

"I can't imagine. I love my assistant job. It doesn't have near the responsibility or demands yours does but I still get to work with kids. It would be nice to have a bigger salary like yours, but I'm not sure if it would compensate for the stress. You teachers have so many people to answer to - your students, their parents, your bosses and colleagues. I admire your dedication."

"Thanks, but if I don't get to bed soon I'll never make it through the day tomorrow. See you on Saturday!"

We took a yoga class together to de-stress. Bernadette had a career, a husband and two children to care for. I was a working, single parent with two children to care for. I had heard that yoga was supposed to be good for people with MS and I liked the simple, gentle poses. The movements got harder and more complicated at the end and I found I lost my sense of focus while trying to push my body. Closing my eyes made balancing more difficult, so I kept them open. I was relieved when the classes ended.

Rachel loved the freedom from small-town living. Her choice of friends concerned me, however, and the day I found a few empty beer bottles and some matches in the attic, I confronted her.

"Rachel, it's the matches that worry me the most. The last thing we need is our house to burn down. I don't want you to go in the unfinished attic any more."

"I don't really like that part of the attic, Mom. It's kind of creepy. I think that's why my friends want to go in there. Maybe we should nail the door shut." Rachel had a tiny ground-floor bedroom with stairs leading to a developed portion of the attic, a kind of loft-like sleeping area. We had removed a small piece of drywall that had been cut as a makeshift door only once to look around at the unfinished portion of the attic, a dirty, dusty cobweb-filled space, so we nailed the door shut. The area was a magnet for kids of that age - it was spooky and cool. When we painted the attic that summer, we sealed the access door with drywall tape, and painted over it. It solved that problem, but fire hazards lurked elsewhere, as I was to discover.

In grade three, we expanded Melissa's trips to the pool by adding a visit to the public library afterwards, which was in the same building. Melissa was growing and gaining weight and I began to notice how tired my back was becoming after an afternoon of her hanging onto my arm for balance and direction. My co-worker noticed the same thing and eventually Melissa got a light, aluminum-framed walker to ease this burden and give her more independence. After much deliberation by an occupational therapist, it was decided the walker would have small wheels in the front only, for safety and stability. It took a few weeks for Mel to accept using the unfamiliar aid, and did not stop occasional falls when she lost her balance, but miraculously she remained unhurt after these tumbles. The walker was usually pulled over sideways, but one day as we entered the library she tripped and went right over the front bar. Melissa laughed. I did not think it was funny. It was dangerous. By the end of the school year, Melissa had a much sturdier metal frame model, with four wheels, a basket, handles with brakes, and a seat.

Winter hit hard in November and our old furnace rattled and clanked as if protesting the overtime work it had to perform in order to keep us warm. The kitchen was freezing and my feet were cold even with thick, warm slippers and a rug under the table where I often sat. Maybe that is why I baked so much - when the oven was on, the kitchen felt much warmer. I sealed up the draughty old windows with plastic and vowed to replace the glass and furnace when I could afford it, hoping the noisy beast would last another winter.

School was closed for two weeks over Christmas, and I could not wait for the break. Not having to rush out the door, plug in the car, shovel snow, scrape ice off the windshield, and battle the cold was wonderful. Sleeping in was even better. The sound of snow blower engines soon became familiar although I preferred the old-fashioned shovel method. It was invigorating and great exercise, but only if I was dressed warmly and not in a hurry. In the dead of winter, when frigid cold descended, it was difficult to decide between walking or driving. My legs protested almost as much as the frozen vehicle and neither were particularly efficient.

One night before Christmas, I talked to Bernadette.

"I really like to go to church on Christmas Eve and I haven't been able to for a long time. Would you be interested in going?" I thought a few Christmas carols and bit of Scripture reading would be perfect to bring meaning to the season.

"You know, Kathy, that might be nice. I'll ask Andy and we'll let you know."

"We could have an early supper together at my place and then walk over to church. It's only half a block. The service is an hour and there's a short play for the children to watch." Except for Rachel, our kids were young, so the seven o'clock service worked well.

We had a wonderful evening together and shared Christmas dinner with our friends at their house the next day.

"What are you doing for New Year's?" I asked. Andy passed the potatoes.

"We haven't decided for sure. I don't have a gig, so we can do whatever we want." Andy was a musician and often sang in local entertainment venues.

Bernadette looked thoughtful as she wiped some spilt juice off the floor. "Sally says she's not doing anything then. We should do something really fun. Do you like fondues?" I clapped my hands in excitement.

"I love fondues! We used to have fondues every year when I was growing up. What kind do you like? We used to have oil fondues, with meat, seafood and veggies to cook and lots of sauces and tempura batter for the veggies. Oh, it was so good." Bernadette laughed.

"Have you ever had cheese fondue? How about chocolate? We could have all three! It is a millennium celebration, after all. I'll talk to Sally and see if she's interested."

I had not had a fondue for years and it was better than I remembered - delicious, savoury, and great fun. Afterwards, we each made a pottery dish out of some clay Sally brought and engraved our name and the date on the bottom. Sally took them home to fire the "works of art" in a kiln. Andy pulled out his guitar and we sang some favourite old tunes. It was a memorable evening shared with close friends.

The girls helped plan our holiday to the Maritimes for the summer of 2000. Rachel did not want to be the only teenager for two weeks. Kelly-Leigh suggested that Rachel might enjoy a stopover in Toronto to spend some time with her nieces, who were about the same age, and Rachel thought this was a "cool" idea. I liked it too. It gave Rachel some independence because she would travel to Toronto on her own and expand her friendship circle. She had withdrawn into her own world of peers and she was now less willing to participate in family time. We arranged to spend time with Kelly-Leigh in New Brunswick, since she had a conference to attend, and she brought Rachel and a niece with her. It was an excellent opportunity to see some of the beautiful east coast and share time with family and friends.

I gave up cross-county skiing at the local golf course that winter because it was either too cold, the snow was sparse, or I was too tired. There was a better place to ski with groomed trails at the local Nordic Ski Center, where I had skied over ten years before and I hoped to take Becky when conditions were just right. We headed out on a warm spring day in late March, during spring break when the kids were out of school. It was precious downtime for me.

"You'll like it much better this time, Becky. Let's take a thermos of hot chocolate, lunch and our sunglasses." Our last experience together at the golf course had been bitterly cold and I was determined to try again.

The trails were icy and hard or wet and slushy where the sun shone - it was a trade-off for warmth. Some ground was beginning to show through in a flat, open section near the lodge. I had forgotten how hilly and steep some of the runs were, even on the shorter novice routes, and the first icy hill with a corner at the end took every ounce of strength in my legs to stay upright. Becky went first and took a tumble at the bottom before the curve. I gritted my teeth and attempted to remain positive.

"Mom, I'm tired," Becky lamented when I caught up to her.

"But we just started! I think that was the biggest hill." I wondered about that.

"You go first this time."

"Okay, but try and keep me in sight," I said as I pushed off with my poles. Between stopping for Becky and dealing with the conditions and rolling terrain, striking any sort of rhythm was almost impossible. It was like skiing on gravel. We came to another big hill.

"I'm not going down that," Becky stated. I gave up after much cajoling, and helped Becky take her skis off so she could walk down. I laughed to myself, remembering the time I had done the same thing as a kid of ten on an intimidating downhill ski slope while my brothers sailed by gleefully.

I forced myself to move forward, quickly sped out of control past Becky, and landed in a twisted heap at the bottom of the treacherous hill.

"Are you okay, Mom?" Becky yelled. I rubbed my sore hip as I stood up, muttering to myself.

"Yeah, I'll live. I hate falling."

"I don't like this trail, Mom, it's too hard." I was secretly beginning to agree. We finished the loop with a few more jarring falls, when it suddenly opened up into a large clearing by the lodge where we had started. I heard the cry of a raven in the distance and slipped on my sunglasses in the dazzling sun.

"Let's have our lunch over there," I said, pointing to the small hut where results were tallied by judges during races. The sun poured in through the glassless viewing windows, and a couple of chairs beckoned. The place was deserted. We wolfed our food down and I stretched out my legs and closed my eyes in the warm midday sun.

~~~~~~

The trail stretched out endlessly, dropping out of sight at the distant horizon. Time stood still as my body repeated the familiar rhythm. Left pole, right leg, right pole, left leg. Back straight, knees bent, breathe, breathe. My thoughts wandered. Suddenly I realized Dave and our friends were nowhere in sight, and I stopped to scan as far as I could see. Pay more attention, Kathy, you're in the backcountry and we haven't seen anyone for miles. Two dots appeared at the far end of the valley, and I sped up as much as possible to catch them. Dave had stopped for a smoke halfway across.

"Go ahead, I'll catch up shortly." I continued and, true to his word, Dave soon caught up and then passed me. Pushing harder, I willed the last few ounces of strength to propel me

forward, eventually reaching the party of three who were
waiting for me. I felt guilty, slowing everyone down.

"Don't wait for me, I need to rest, and then I'll catch up."
Liar, you're getting slower each moment. As soon as I
stopped, my toes froze, and I forced myself to continue. Left
pole, right leg, right pole, left leg. Concentrate, focus. I came
to a section that followed a frozen riverbed and wound
through stunted lodge pole pines, and recognized the last
stretch of the journey. I was so tired.

~~~~~~

"Mommmm! Earth to Mom, did you even hear what I
said?" Becky shook my arm impatiently as I brought my
thoughts back to the present.

"Sorry, I was day-dreaming. What did you say?"

"Can we go home soon? I don't like the icy ski trail."

"Me neither. I think I might have some bruises from
those hard falls. Are you okay?" I started packing up
our things.

"I'm fine. Can we go?" So much for recreation with
my kid! At least we gave it a shot, and the sun softened
not only the snow, but my outlook as well. My memory
of the backcountry ski trip in Jasper National Park,
when Rachel was small and Becky had not been born
left me wondering how I could have brushed aside the
exhaustion. I had not even thought of it until now, over
ten years later.

~~~~~~

By June, all the details of our trip to the Maritimes
had been arranged. Becky and I caught our plane to
Nova Scotia in early July, in the late evening. I thought
we would sleep for most of the overnight flight, but a
delay in Calgary altered flight plans and instead we had
a five-hour unexpected stopover.

It was a very long night. Becky was overtired and
could not sit still. Around 2 am, the cleaning crew

started vacuuming and collecting garbage. I wanted to scream at the janitors, but Becky finally fell asleep to the whirr of machines, so I stifled my outrage and attempted to sleep. What would happen if I slept through the departure? Bewildered, we barely made it to our plane, turning the wrong way in the huge airport and getting lost. We dozed on and off during the flight, and I could not wait for a real bed.

My smart, capable girlfriend had booked a hotel for us near the airport where we landed in Nova Scotia, and took us there in a rented minivan, certain we needed to rest before heading out to explore the next day. She was right. It helped tremendously and we were revived enough to continue.

Kelly-Leigh, her niece Martine, Rachel, Becky and I piled into the spacious van the following morning and drove northward, turning west towards New Brunswick where we passed through Truro. Colourful flowers clustered in ditches beside the highways and I recognized the tall pea-like plants as lupines, much taller than any I had seen. The flowers were introduced to the Maritimes from the Mediterranean as ornamental, quickly escaping the confines of a few gardens and eventually growing wild, to be admired by locals and visitors alike.

We came to Amherst, and crossed the border into New Brunswick. The two-lane highway changed to a single lane and we found ourselves in quaint, rural communities that dotted the Cumberland Basin and Petitcodiac River, as we followed the road up to Moncton. Coastal fog had descended upon the area as we changed direction towards Hopewell Cape. The hilly countryside with meandering rivers led us across covered wooden bridges and we stopped to admire their old world charm and the surrounding hills. We could smell the salty ocean air. Inland heat dissipated as we neared "Hopewell Rocks."

A short, sloping trail led us down to never ending stairs that allowed visitors to access the beach and walk directly around the huge towering rocks. Described as "giant flower pots," they were the legacy of 300 million years of the earth's development. Sea caves had been created from a salt conglomerate, formed under tremendous pressure.

Kelly-Leigh and the girls raced on ahead, while I stopped and rested on the landings, taking my time, slow and steady. Stunted trees and vegetation grew on the tops of some of the tallest rocks, which resembled pointy mushroom tops that created a fairy-tale setting. Archways had been carved between the massive structures. Water lapped the shores, and the most weathered, gently curved rocks sat like stepping-stones offering a path out to sea, where mist hung, almost touching the water and obliterating any further view.

I caught up to the group of intrepid explorers.

"Hey, you guys, I mean gals, I want your picture with one of these interesting rocks behind you." I took a fabulous shot of the four smiling friends, crouched together, fog creating a solid gray backdrop for the rock profiles etched into the sky. The highest tides in the world had not destroyed the rocks.

The next day we followed the highway along the ocean to Fundy National Park. Becky and I walked leisurely along the trail while Kelly-Leigh and the older girls set off at a faster pace. The coniferous trees were scraggly, moss-covered mammoths and the forest floor was a mass of shrubs, plants and decaying fallen trees. We inhaled salty ocean air, heard water rushing and slamming up against rock, but the ocean was hidden from view.

Travelling southwest, we drove parallel to the Bay of Fundy and stopped in Saint Martins, a pretty fishing village beside the ocean. We inquired about whale watching. The fog had cleared, it was windy on the water but to our disappointment, there were no whales to be seen, so we continued to our destination, Saint John, to spend the next few days.

"Do you girls want to go to the children's program offered tomorrow? Bowling is planned - that could be kind of fun." Kelly-Leigh winked at me. I was dreaming about a few hours of free time while the kids and their aunt were busy, as Kelly-Leigh's days were booked up with the veterinary convention.

"Bowling, bowling, let's go bowling," Becky chanted. It sounded as though I had tomorrow off "mom" duties. What a treat!

"What are you gonna do, Mom?"

"Oh, I don't know, maybe I'll be really bored and lonely." I smiled broadly at my friend. "I'm just kidding, Becky, it'll be nice to have some free time to wander around the city exploring some of the beautiful old buildings I saw glimpses of as we drove in."

Our hotel was on the edge of the harbour, and, after dropping the kids off the next morning, I followed an escalator up a level and discovered a corridor filled with shops and glass walkways that provided glimpses of the city. I passed an entry to the Maritime Museum and made a note to visit before we left.

The streets rose from sea level and I could pick out most of the landmarks, so I tucked the little street map into my pocket. The architecture of the first church was a combination of stone, wood, elaborate carving and ornate glass. I slipped inside and marvelled at the intricate detail. Each building I viewed was similar, some smaller and less regal, but all were charming and well cared for. The shops had an array of souvenirs. I bought a few postcards and sat on a bench to rest, not exhausted but suddenly starving. After a late lunch, I realized I had left my jacket somewhere in my earlier travels. I was certain that if I retraced my steps, it would be there. I had earned the jacket as a member of the Fire Department, so it was a favourite, but I had no luck finding it and sadly returned to the hotel in time to pick up the kids. I flopped down in a chair and shared a drink with my friend, tired from the extra walking.

The girls and I spent the following day together, exploring the museum and sights in the area. In the evening, Kelly-Leigh joined us as we shared delicious food and time together, and the week passed all too quickly.

Our friends David and Helene picked us up in a vintage 1951 Studebaker, lovingly restored and proudly driven. It had been six years since we had seen each other.

"Oh my gosh, is that you, Rachel? Good thing your mom keeps us updated with pictures or I wouldn't have recognized you." The baby and young girl that Helene had known had grown into a young woman, an insecure teenager who related to friends her own age. She felt shy and uncomfortable around adults.

"And Becky, you look a lot like your sister. You weren't even born when we moved."

It was so good to see my friend with whom I had spent ten years of my life sharing laughter, tears, good times, hard times, conversation and most of all encouragement. The bond remained strong despite distance and time. I hugged her hard.

We spent two wonderful weeks together.

"What's the name of the town again?" Becky asked.

"Parrsboro. It's where I grew up, Becky. My mother

still lives there, a few houses away from ours." David was proud of his heritage and was a knowledgeable host and tour guide. They opened their home and spent time and energy showing us the best of their beautiful province.

"I can't wait to see your property and the town I've heard so much about." It had been the couple's dream to own land and a homestead after years of living in an apartment.

It was lovely. The property was huge, with a detached garage, greenhouse, and sprawling lawns and gardens.

"How old is the house, David?"

"It was built around 1895. It's an ongoing project of repair and restoration. Keeps me out of trouble, though." David was a retired engineer, and Helene worked at the school across the street. Beside their property sat another heritage building, with a steeply pitched gable roof and rows of tall glass windows, which had humble beginnings in 1885 as a Presbyterian church.

It was much cooler than I had expected and it was rainy for the first few days. I could not get warm, and had trouble sleeping with a restless five-year old. Finally, the rain quit and we ventured out on a day trip towards Cape D'or, a spit of land jutting into the Bay of Fundy, where ocean, rocks and rolling green hills met. A lighthouse stood on the edge of the cliffs and we wandered around soaking in the warmth. I took lots of pictures. It was beautiful.

We stopped at several points along the route, where the road wound through the land and often brought us within sight of the calm, blue ocean. Lighthouses, cliffs and red rocks filled the space beside the vast expanse of water. The Red Rocks were famous in the Cumberland County, an area of Nova Scotia rich in history and resources.

"Do you girls like strawberries?" Helene asked when we got home. The girls both nodded quickly. "Would you like to go picking tomorrow? I know of a perfect spot where we can pick as much as we like and bring berries home for the freezer."

"Where is it?" Becky demanded.

"Don't worry, it's not a long drive like we did today. It's close to here, and we'll be home by lunch before it gets too hot. We'll take a bunch of buckets and pick for as long as we like."

"Can we eat strawberries while we pick?" Becky's eyes lit up.

"I think so. Last year we hauled home twenty–two pounds and had strawberries in the winter." Helene smiled at the memory.

"It's been years since I've been to a u-pick fruit farm. The girls will love it." I could not wait to eat big, juicy strawberries in the warm east coast sun.

The next day we were on our hands and knees wearing sun block and hats, filling containers and our mouths. The hills were covered with rows of strawberry plants and the low-lying, dark green vines stretched out across the field, the air thick with fragrant fruit, buzzing insects and the sweat of our labour. Taste buds stimulated by the delicate, delicious berries were soon saturated and bellies filled to satisfaction. Further work continued at home to wash and cut off the leafy tops in preparation for the freezer. It was strawberry heaven.

Rachel kept disappearing into her guest bedroom for hours and our hosts were concerned.

"Why doesn't she come and visit with us?" they asked, puzzled.

"Well," I said, "it seems to be part of a phase she's going through, being uncomfortable around adults when there are no other kids her age." I made a note to talk to Rachel privately about trying to be more sociable.

We planned a day trip to Prince Edward Island and had another ride in the Studebaker. David relayed bits of history and trivia as he drove northward. I tried to catch Rachel's eye several times but she was absorbed in a book.

"Rachel, look at the beautiful old houses in this town, and the neat little shops. There's a tiny school that reminds me of the Bryan School." Rachel glanced up and nodded.

"Uh-huh. Nice." She returned to reading. The pastoral towns surrounded by farmland and trees stretched for miles. I soaked in the tranquil setting.

"We're coming up to the bridge soon," David announced. Becky pressed her nose against the glass, and I twisted my neck for a better view as the offensive stink of farm manure reached my nose. The strong ocean breeze carried it away quickly.

Confederation Bridge was completed in 1997 and links New Brunswick to Prince Edward Island. At 12.9 kilometres, it's the longest bridge (over ice-covered waters) in the world and an amazing engineering feat. Before I had a chance to appreciate the magnitude, we were driving on it, and it was only when we stopped at the other end that I saw pier after pier carrying the bridge across the water. The concrete walls (girders) on either side of the four lanes did not allow for a close-up view of the ocean and it soon felt like any old highway. It was not possible to see the huge, concrete supports that disappeared into the ocean as we were driving, but the postcard I bought gave a stunning aerial view that conveyed the vast length of the bridge. It was impressive.

We drove to the east side of the island, stopping at the

"Anne of Green Gables" heritage site and went on to find a legendary east coast white sandy beach, Cavendish. The sand was soft, fine and dune-like in some sections and the ocean was warm with gentle, lapping waves. It was hot, a great day for the beach. Becky and Rachel built sand castles near a shallow pool that made an ideal place for sculpting. I watched indulgently as they ran into the ocean screaming, emerging with dripping bodies. They collapsed into the soft sand, rolling around like sugar-cookie dough that is dipped in sugar, sand sticking to their warm bodies. The adults relaxed on big beach towels, ventured into the waves for fun, and combed the shoreline for souvenir seashells. We returned to Parrsboro in the evening, satiated with the glories of the east coast. The cool evening breeze off the shore of the Minas Basin lulled us to sleep.

Most of the access to the water was rocky. I cautiously picked my way across the beaches we explored, conscious of my slowness, concentrating on planting the first foot firmly before lifting the other off shifting rock. The soft sand had not been a problem but the hard, pebble-like rock was much less forgiving.

Helene's creative side appealed to the girls and they spent hours in a bright sunroom with scissors, paper, ribbon and a variety of craft material including beeswax, seashells and local rocks. The polished rocks felt smooth and cool, as did some of the weathered, shiny seashells. Rachel was in her element.

"Do you girls like Ferris-wheels, roller coasters and fast rides? How about cotton candy and snow cones? I know you like clowns, how about haunted houses and silly guessing games?" Helene's hobby was clowning, and she had taken Becky with her on a town parade when we had first arrived. Rachel put her scissors down.

"I love fairs. We have one in our town called Derby Days." Rachel was usually gone for hours when the travelling carnival came to our town in June, and the novelty of such an event had not worn off. She stood up, craft forgotten.

"I thought we could go tonight for a bit of fun. It's just a mile or so down the road." Helene pulled a couple of small containers off the shelf. "I have a surprise for you. Rachel, can you help Becky count this?" she said as she handed Rachel the jars.

"Wow, look at all the twoonies!" The kids dumped the coins on the table.

"I've been saving for a while so I could treat you girls to some spending money for the fair."

I looked at my good friend in admiration at her forethought and generosity. She was a special lady with a heart for children, especially mine.

It was a typical small town carnival and the girls were drawn into the excitement. In no time, Rachel was trailing around with a couple of local kids her own age. Rachel's week with us was almost over because she was scheduled to fly back to Toronto and spend the last week of holidays with Kelly-Leigh's family. Her aloofness had caused some tension in the house already, so a full two weeks would have been too much for all concerned. I felt torn. I did not want my friends to be hurt, but I also wanted Rachel to feel comfortable and enjoy the time we had together.

We continued to enjoy Maritime hospitality, through David and Helene's dedication to showing us a variety of sights, sounds and tastes in their beloved province. The weather was typically coastal – warm balmy days, cool calm evenings, and hotter inland. David was especially excited about some ships that were scheduled to arrive in Halifax during our last week of visiting, and we planned a trip to the capital city of Nova Scotia before catching our plane home. He handed me a brochure.

"Here's some info on the ships with some scheduled events. I've been looking forward to this for quite a while. The last time we had Tall Ships visit Halifax was 1984. We'll stay with our good friends about five blocks from the harbour, so we can walk and take in as much as we want."

I scanned the write-up.

"This July 19-24, more than 150 majestic barques, brigantines, clippers and schooners, from 22 countries around the world, will visit our historic oceanside city as part of a four-month international competition billed as the 'Race of the Century.'"

I looked at a picture of a full rigged sailing ship and realized how fortunate we were.

To get there, we climbed up and away from the ocean, through lush green hills, agricultural land and historic towns, turning south towards Halifax and the Atlantic Ocean. David and Helene's friends were retired. They welcomed us to their home in the heart of the city. It was odd to have a residential street mixed with businesses, shops and restaurants, but the four-level home had a small backyard garden oasis that was a lovely, private escape.

I had trouble sleeping in the hot, breezeless room on the top floor and the heat of the city seeped into my pores. The following day we walked downhill to the water where masses of people met in anticipation of the first Tall Ship arrivals. The harbour was alive with excitement and activity. Smells - ethnic food cooking, fish stands, salt water, suntan lotion, smoke and gasoline fumes that tickled my nose. Sounds - music thick with drums, rhythm, voices, horns, sirens, and the rush of water against manmade walls. Sights - colourful clothing, bodies of all shapes and sizes, skin colour, background, and of course, ships docked alongside the wharf, magnificent, huge and dominating the sky. I held Becky's hand tightly in the sea of humanity.

Haphazard planks forced me to slow my pace and look down more often than I wanted to. There was so much to see. It was exhilarating and exhausting at the same time. After several hours of touring the area, we decided to head back for a late supper.

As we trudged up the hill, my feet felt as though they were glued to the hot pavement and I grimaced and wiped the sweat off my forehead. My left leg refused to follow the right and without realizing it, I was limping from one block to the next and scanning the horizon for the next concrete ledge where I could stop to rest. David carried Becky on his shoulders at the beginning and then Helene took a turn and led her along as I trailed further and further behind. I arrived exhausted, incapable of more than sitting and drinking a cold beer.

"You should have told us it was too much," Helene said in concern.

"I didn't know that would happen," I answered, frustrated.

We spent the rest of our time taking in various tourist attractions, including visiting the lovely City Gardens that stretched on for blocks, touring the famous Halifax Citadel National Historic Site, which offered spectacular views of the harbour and Tall Ships, and sharing culinary delights together. Taking no chances, we drove to anything that involved walking and I appreciated the care and concern of my hosts. When most of the Tall

Ships had arrived, we spent some time touring, photographing and marvelling at the complex designs. I rested on benches whenever available, stayed out of the sun and had no more weak-leg syndrome. It had scared me into awareness and action.

Home was a refuge for the remainder of the summer. I took the training wheels off Becky's new two-wheeled bicycle and we walked around the corner to the high school sports field. With one hand on a handlebar and the other on the seat, I managed to launch her down the faintest incline on the grass where she peddled like mad and stayed upright for short time. We did this over and over until we both fell on the grass, exhausted.

"You did it, Becky! You're riding the bike on your own! Yahoo, we can go bike riding together."

"But I need to practise more first, Mom."

"I know, but once you practise you'll find riding on pavement a lot easier."

We rode bikes together for the next four years, while Becky got stronger and I became weaker. I did not care because I had the wind in my face and the scenery racing by. Eventually, I needed a toe clip for the left side to prevent my weak left foot from sliding off the pedal, but my balance remained undisturbed as I pedalled on.

At the end of August, we started attending a Sunday morning service at a nearby church. My new friend, Kristin, whose husband was a pastor, encouraged me and I decided to give it try since I had never had a chance to belong to a church. Christianity was a bit of a mystery to me, even though I thought I held many Christian values and knew I believed in God. The girls and I were invited to their home for dinner and I was nervous and curious, never having met a pastor before. To my relief, it was informal and relaxed. Their children went to the school where I worked and Becky and their daughter were only two years apart in age. They struck up an instant friendship. Over a delicious meal, which we all seemed to enjoy equally, I fired some questions at Daren about his chosen vocation.

"So what does a person have to do to become a pastor?" It seemed to me you had to be born into this dramatic role or to be someone important at the very least.

"Well, I obtained a degree in Theology, and then began working in a church in Alberta." He smiled. "It wasn't that hard to get started."

"So, post-secondary education, like any other profession. Did you have to have any formal training before that?"

Daren shook his head. "Not really. Every profession has its pre-requisites, but it was nothing unusual."

It was that simple. Well, that blew a hole in all my pre-conceptions. "Do we need a membership, do we have to join something, pay some money?" I asked a bit puzzled.

"No, Kathy, you can just start coming to our church any time you like." The phone rang, and Daren excused himself. I looked over at Kristin, who sat quietly.

"Maybe we'll start coming when school starts. I had no idea it was so simple."

Kristin smiled. "Anytime; it would be great to have you there."

Daren came back in shorts and a T-shirt. "I'm off to play racquet-ball. Nice to meet you." And he was gone. Kristin and I cleared the dishes. The doorbell rang and her son disappeared into the backyard. It was a lot like our house - a bit chaotic and filled with energy.

I felt rested when we returned to school in the fall, but within a month I was chronically tired. Living from weekend to weekend, break to break, I would rest, sleep and build up my energy for the next onslaught of activity. Sometimes I would manage fine and even enjoy it, but it was becoming more difficult. I went to talk to a psychologist about my fears. How would I cope with all the responsibilities? I still felt strong and fit but found it hard to accept the new limitations my body was placing upon me. I was not used to being restricted in activity. The weakness that had hit me in Nova Scotia had been frightening. It gave me a new perspective. Keeping fit was not going to be easy or a solution to my fluctuating energy because determination would only see me so far.

Kristin invited me to weekly Bible study at her house. I thought this was a good way to learn and get some of my questions answered. I learned that in my weakness, God is strong, and I did not have to do this on my own. I had a good support system and God was joining as the team leader. It was just what I needed.

~~~~~~

Rachel was in grade nine and challenged me with her erratic behaviour. She did not really like school but dragged herself out of bed most mornings. The emotional outbursts, anger and tears (part of adolescence, I was told) was draining to live with for a single mom trying to keep things on an even keel. My oldest daughter was insecure and sensitive, falling asleep at odd hours and constantly on the phone.

One evening I baked brownies after Becky had gone to bed and disappeared into my bedroom while they were baking to prepare for the next workday. There was a loud, anguished cry from Rachel's bedroom. *Thump, crash, thump.* Rachel had slipped a few times on the narrow stairs and I told myself for the millionth time I needed to carpet the slippery wood surface to prevent further accidents. *Bang, crash, wack.* Rachel slammed a door. I had threatened to take her bedroom door off the hinges a few times but had never followed through. I investigated.

"Rachel, are you okay?" A wail came from within.

"Go away. I just want to be by myself." She started crying louder than ever.

"Rachel, sshhhhh, you'll wake Becky," I reprimanded uselessly. The howling continued and I heard the bathroom door slam.

I wandered into the kitchen to get a piece of brownie, to discover the pan was nowhere in sight. Following my instinct, I went into Rachel's room and carefully climbed the attic stairs. Instead of brownie, a strong smell of burning candles reached my nose. In fact, I could smell smoke and gasped when I saw flames coming from the lampshade that sat on a side table underneath the four-foot ceiling. I scrambled across the carpeted floor on my hands and knees and blew out the candle. Grabbing a towel, I smothered the lamp and looked down at the singed carpet. Spilt wax was warm to my touch. A section of ceiling above the lampshade was black with smoke and the room stank of acrid fumes. I opened the window forcefully, as the adrenaline that rushed through my body subsided like the ebb of seawater drawn back to its source. I snatched the brownie that sat precariously at the edge of the night table and headed downstairs.

Bang, bang, bang. "Rachel, open the door. I need to talk to you." She was still locked in the bathroom, crying.

I went to the kitchen and cut myself some brownie, sitting and thinking about the best way to handle this. No more candles, for sure. My instinct told me that attics, candles and teenagers were a bad combination and my firefighter training told me it was potentially deadly. How was I going to get the message across effectively? Telling, talking and lecturing would not work, just as grounding and punishment would likely not, so I grabbed a piece of paper and decided to appeal to Rachel's theatrical side. Drama queen, meet drama mom.

In large capital letters, I wrote, **"FIRE KILLS."** Underneath in small print I outlined the plan:

"No more candles. A fire started (while you were having a meltdown on the phone, no pun intended), because you left burning candles unattended in the attic. Go see for yourself."

On a whim, I lit a match and burnt the edges of the paper lightly. It gave a dramatic flair to the note, exactly what was needed, and I carried it into Rachel's room and placed it on the stairs. It was late and I went to bed, not really sleepy, but tired. Eventually, doors were opened and I strained to hear. The stairs creaked. Silence. I pictured her reading the note and coming to me with excuses and apologies, but I waited in vain. I heard some muffled noises in her room and drifted off, dreaming of huge shooting flames and sirens in the distance.

Before I left for work the next morning, I yelled to Rachel at the bottom of the stairs.

"Aren't you going to class? It's eight o'clock."

"Huh? I don't have to be there until second period," she said in a muffled voice.

"Okay, you know your schedule. I'll see you after school."

"Uh-huh."

I wondered all day if Rachel would avoid me, but after school, she cruised past me in the kitchen with an armload of stuff. She came back with a half-filled garbage bag.

"I'm throwing out all my candles," she said as she

stopped and opened the bag. I saw an assortment of partially burnt candles and nodded at her approvingly. She disappeared out the back door. I heard a thud as the bag was thrown into the garbage dumpster.

"Wow. A good move, I think."

"Yeah, I'm sorry. I had a really upsetting phone call and forgot about everything else." Rachel grabbed an old cloth and some cleaning solution from under the sink. "I threw the lampshade away, and I'll clean up what I can."

"It's actually a good thing you took the brownie upstairs, or I wouldn't have gone up to the attic. I think you understand how serious it could have been." Rachel nodded, and I was relieved she was acting responsibly. It had scared me, and maybe scared her too. Good. We needed action, not words.

NINE

"There are strange things done
in the midnight sun…"
~ Robert Service ~

I spent half my workday assisting Melissa, who was in grade four, and the other half in kindergarten, which I loved. The children were so funny, very sweet, and very young. Everything was new to them - the classroom, the teacher, the routine, craft time, structured play time and special activity time that included trips to the gym for games and exercise, the computer lab for "lessons" on the computer, and other events that came up from time to time.

Getting to know the children was interesting and by Christmas, I could see personality types already. There were shy, quiet ones, loud, aggressive ones, cooperative, uncooperative, happy, cheerful social ones and loners. Most liked attention, playing and interacting. I enjoyed getting down on the carpet at their level and playing with blocks, puzzles, and dolls, as well as at a variety of "play stations," such as the sandbox. I sat in the little chairs with them during snack time, and learned about their families and ideas.

The students sat on the carpet each day and gathered round the teacher for discussion and story-time. This gave me a chance to prep supplies and ready equipment for use. One day the teacher asked me if I would like to read the story, which sent a little shiver down my spine. I was nervous with twenty pairs of eyes on me but soon forgot about the attention as my enthusiasm in making the story as entertaining as possible took over. The kids listened closely at the start and as their attention started to wander, I changed my voice, hammed it up a little, or stopped to ask a question. Stories with repetitive lines were the best, as the children could not wait to join in shouting out the line or word they knew best.

When a student came to sit close to me or placed their little hand in mine to walk down the long hallway, my heart and tiredness melted. Each child was unique, full of trust and curious about everything.

Melissa, who was chronologically in grade four and treated as such, was really at this level and it gave me tons of ideas to improve her individual programming. The gap was growing. Even though she was physically at par with kids her age, the remainder of her life skills fell far behind, especially communication. I brought her to kindergarten a few times and she was happy to crawl around on the carpet and play, but the kindergarten kids stared and wanted to know what was wrong. She was so much bigger than they were, and did not fit in.

On the other end of the scale, in grade four it was a waste of time for us to stay in the classroom where students were learning advanced math skills, reading novels and building science experiments that were far beyond anything she could attain. Integration was not the solution as I had once thought it could be. There were no simple answers, and we did what we could to improve her quality of life. She was not unhappy, and for that, I was grateful.

We were working on a communication system to help

Melissa convey specific needs and wants to those around her. It was called Picture Exchange Communication System, PECS, and Melissa's alternate aide and I had been trained in how to develop and put the program into use at school. It was very confusing at first. Breaking communication down into step-by-step, simple concepts in the form of pictures was not as easy as it sounded.

The program had a number of levels, each one building on the previous. A speech therapist from the local Health Unit helped us get started by using a stiff plastic binder and a few basic pictures.

"You'll need to laminate the pictures you want to start with, since they'll be used over and over, and hold them in place in the binder with Velcro. You can easily buy strips of sticky-back Velcro and order more pages, then shrink and laminate more pictures as you go. We usually start with larger pictures, and decrease the size over time in order to expand the number of pictures used." The speech pathologist placed a picture of a school bus on the front of the binder to illustrate. "You, and eventually Melissa, would put this picture on the front of the binder when she is ready to catch the bus." She pulled the picture off and placed a picture of a sandwich, apple and yogurt on the cover. "When Melissa learns how to use this effectively, she would put this picture on the cover to show and tell she is hungry."

"Can we use more than one picture?" my partner asked. We had an inventory of hundreds of pictures to choose from, in a huge binder, universal to all using the program.

"Eventually you can use several pictures, but for now we'll concentrate on one at a time."

When we thought we were ready, we brought Melissa into the room. Shirley and I illustrated the picture exchange between each other to give Melissa an idea of how it worked. Melissa smiled sweetly at us, but when we first tried to engage her participation, she just sat there. I stood behind her and guided her hand, showing her how to move the picture. It took a while, but she got it and soon started using the pictures herself. Her binder went with her everywhere, and one of the goals was for her to be able to communicate with anyone this way. It was a great step forward. If only we could keep up with her physical needs.

Melissa had grown almost as big as Shirley, who was barely five feet tall. Even though we had a heavier walker, Melissa still needed physical assistance to get in and out of a desk or chair, move around in a bathroom, get up off the floor, board the bus, and get dressed and changed for swimming.

"You know, Kathy, I don't think I can handle this next year." Shirley had been with Melissa for three years.

"I have to start thinking about that too. It's getting harder; Mel's so big now."

"My back can't take much more," Shirley said, rubbing her lower back.

We even had an elevator installed for handicapped people to get to the upper wing of classrooms. I really enjoyed working with Mel, even though it wore me out some days, but was considering staying with her another year. The school owned a wheelchair that sat in the main entrance hallway, and we had been told we were welcome to use it. I understood Melissa needed to get exercise and her parents wanted her to remain mobile, but sometimes there was a lot of distance to cover and it might come in handy.

Many of the special needs students in the school system had moderate to severe behaviour problems and even though the physical challenges were minor, I found short stints with these kids far more exhausting than working with disabled students.

One day I watched in disbelief as a young boy in grade two attacked his teacher, kicking and biting her in a rage. Some of the aides I knew endured this kind of behaviour on a regular basis. It was frightening. How could these children be part of a public school system? It was not fair to anyone – the teachers, aides, students affected in the classroom, and even the disruptive child. Was inclusion of all children the right solution?

Spring break was cold and snowy – it made it easy to stay home and relax. Neither of the girls seemed to mind so I spent hours in my room, reading and sleeping. Students from the grade-five classroom I worked in had been writing limericks and it reminded me of how much I liked poetry. In a rush of inspiration, I picked up my pen and wrote alongside the kids. Creativity flowed all around me. There was further encouragement from some poetry books a teacher had ordered from the Scholastic Book Club for her students, and I had borrowed a few to take home and look over during the week off.

At my house, I dug out the "Norton Anthology of English Literature" that I had kept from a university English class I had taken many years ago. The names Wordsworth, Blake, and Coleridge caught my eye as I turned the flimsy pages, and my carefully pencilled notations in the margins of "The Rime of the Ancient Mariner" reminded me I that my writing of poetry had been sporadic at best and my passion for writing had long been abandoned.

As a child, my father's enjoyment of poetry was apparent in what he read to us – *Winnie the Pooh, The Tales of Christopher Robin,* and *Dr. Seuss,* and when we got older, he would recite by heart Robert Service's "The

Cremation of Sam McGee." Kelly-Leigh still remembers my Dad turning the lights down low, lighting his pipe and entrancing us with his rendition of a frozen stiff Sam.

> "The Northern Lights have seen queer sights,
> But the queerest they ever did see
> Was the night on the marge of Lake Lebarge
> I cremated Sam McGee."

In the warm glow of Dad's pipe, we could just imagine Sam warming up in the derelict "Alice May" furnace.

In grade eight, an influential, passionate English teacher had encouraged my love of writing in both poetry and prose. It was my favourite subject all through school and here I was again in a school, still a student at heart, thirty years later.

Metaphors, similes, couplets and personification. I wrote down the definitions. I had never heard of onomatopoeia - how do you pronounce that? "A word that makes the sound of the action it describes." Like hiss, honk and whoosh. What was assonance? "Repetition of vowel sounds, like meet and heat." I made a list, and laughed when I barely knew half the terms. I discovered I used these figures of speech instinctively in my writing and soon forgot about the definitions. It was like reading the Bible - you can have a passion for God but not know the Scriptures by heart.

I wrote a poem about what it felt like to have multiple sclerosis, my little secret from the world. Even though my life was full and busy, being single was sometimes lonely, and I explored these feelings in a poem filled with personification and opposites. My understanding of Christianity was growing and I wrote a poem about angels using the five senses of sight, sound, taste, touch and smell, and found inspiration pouring through me. I wrote poetry about nature, mountains, cats and friendship. The pain from my failed marriage poured out on the page in fourteen verses entitled "Different This Time." Writing unleashed pent-up emotions, a dam breaking with furious power, eventually spreading out into calmer waters.

Spring was a renewing time for me. After the long, harsh cold of winter, the promise of warmth, growth and lazy summer days was tantalizing and improved motivation. It seemed the birds and trees agreed with me and even our two cats appreciated the freedom of a less hostile great outdoors, judging by the number of times I opened the door to let them out. No wonder people installed special "cat doors."

The doctor's office called.

"I have an appointment time for you, Kathy. The neurologist would like to see you on June 5, at 1 pm, if you can make it." I grabbed a calendar and checked the dates.

"I'll have to see if I can get that day off work. Can I let you know by tomorrow?" I would book the day off for medical or personal leave. It was important. My health counted for a lot. I used to buy into society's message "health is everything" but in facing MS, I saw there were a huge number of people out there, young and old, without the best of health and they were coping, surviving and even leading productive lives. I was lucky enough to be working, raising two children and happy. I coped with the ups and downs of life like most people. I felt joy, elation and satisfaction tempered with frustration, sadness and sometimes anger.

Modern medicine could not offer people like me a cure for chronic illness, but that did not mean that working in the traditional sense was the only way to live. I tried to expand my thinking and make room for an uncertain future. My Bible study group offered a new perspective that health is not everything and I started to see the world in a different light.

Moisture was lacking in the ground in May after an unusually dry spring so forest fires were burning around the province. My forestry days seemed long ago. Our front lawn resembled a moonscape of uneven, desiccated terrain sucked dry by the huge, unkempt spruce trees that dropped needles onto the lawn and leeched the soil of nutrients. The feeble attempts I had made at cutting the lowest branches off the massive trees made little difference, and when my neighbour took pity on me and helped cut away the dead foliage, he attempted to rejuvenate my lawn by aerating it. The new picture windows at the front of our house did little to improve the dullness.

When a neighbour with a trucking business offered to cut some or all of the trees down, I was ready. It was a matter of when and how many trees. Six tall spruces bordered the edge of our property. I valued the privacy created by the trees but missed the sunlight. The deep roots were destroying the lawn. A month passed without any action and my attention turned to other events.

Smoke from nearby forest fires was lingering in the air and combined with sudden blasts of pulp-mill odour, it was unappealing to spend time outdoors in the neighbourhood. My friend Rick phoned me one day at the end of May.

"Have you heard the bad news, Kathy? John Graham was killed yesterday fighting in a forest fire. He and the pilot both died." Rick's forestry background kept him connected in the world of Forests, Lands and Wildlife. I was shocked.

"But he just got settled in Grande Prairie and was living out his dream of flying as a Bird-dog officer. That's unbelievable; such a tragedy. What exactly happened?" This was a man I had worked for and alongside on a professional, volunteer and friendship basis for almost ten years. I had a deep respect for John.

"I guess they got too close to the heat and the drafts created by the inferno pulled them in. There are a number of fires burning out of control right now in the province."

"Yeah, I caught that on recent news, but nothing about this. Keep me posted on plans for a funeral, will you?" I hung up, and sat stunned by the news.

Rick and I both took the day off work to drive up to Grande Prairie and attend the funeral. John left behind his wife, a grown daughter and a teenage daughter. He was fifty-nine years old. The only consolation was that John died doing something he loved. The huge funeral with men and women in full Forestry uniform and planes flying overhead told the story of just how much he was respected and would be missed. I wrote a poem and tucked it inside the bereavement card. It helped my tears to flow.

~~~~~~

Back at work, I barely had time to settle in before I had to make yet another trip to Edmonton to meet the neurologist. He introduced himself and a second young doctor who smiled at me as he shook my hand.

"Hi, Kathy, this is Dr. Gabriel. He's with me today to observe, as part of his training. Have a seat and we'll go over your history." We covered some basics and confirmed previous findings.

"Can we have you walk from one end of the room to the other, turn, and come back?"

I tried to relax and walk as normally as possible. The

151

familiar catch in my left leg was causing a subtle limp, barely noticeable to the casual observer but to me a harsh, glaring spotlight – look, there is something wrong with her. How could people not notice my wonky walk, or were they just too polite to say?

"Can you remove your shoes and sit up on the examination table?" The young doctor used a few instruments to test reflexes, sensation, strength and vision while the neurologist scribbled madly on a clipboard.

Extensive discussion ensued about various treatment options. The focus was on four "disease modifying drugs" that slowed the progression of the disease and were the most current treatment available for relapsing-remitting multiple sclerosis in 2001. We discussed cost, insurance, injections and information sources for me to explore before making any decisions. I found a wealth of material on the Internet, through the MS Society and by contacting people with the disease who were using a drug treatment of this type. What seemed straightforward quickly became overwhelming with so much information and so many people involved in the decision - my insurance company, employer, doctors, nurses and ultimately, myself. I did not have a spouse for feedback and my kids needed me as their mother, not as someone they had to take care of. That was the decisive factor – I would do whatever was necessary to remain an active parent even if it meant poking a needle in myself every day.

Some big hurdles had to be to overcome. Would the insurance company fund my use of the drug? Could I continue working while on this medication? How would I handle self-injection? How much would it really help? What would my children think?

I started by applying to the insurance company for

coverage of this expensive drug, filling out pages of forms, collecting letters from doctors, and coordinating recommendations from the neurologist. The process was underway in early June.

While waiting for the insurance company to determine coverage, I collected information. The local chapter of the MS Society was glad to send me what literature was available on current drugs used in the treatment of multiple sclerosis and a trip to the library gave me some reference books that were helpful. At home, on our personal computer, the Internet had a vast resource of information and I was quickly bogged down. I enlisted Rachel's help.

"Rachel, how do I find out about this specific drug? It will take me days to read through all this stuff I've found." Rachel knew a lot more about computers than I did. She laughed and knelt down beside me as she gripped the mouse.

"Look, Mom, you just click in this box and type the words you want to know about." In no time, I had what I needed.

"Thanks, Rachel. I think I need to learn some computer basics."

"Yes, that would be a good idea." Rachel and Becky were miles ahead of me in knowledge and understanding – it was time for me to gain some skill. My workplace was one area to start and maybe I could manage an evening course. I had just completed my teacher's aide certificate by correspondence and I was encouraged by the ease at which I finished the program.

I learned that interferons are proteins produced naturally by the human body to fight viral infections. In other words, they do what their name implies - they interfere with the damage caused by the virus. Multiple sclerosis is an autoimmune disease, which means the body gets messages confused. Instead of protecting itself, it does the opposite and attacks the central nervous system (CNS; the brain, spinal cord and optic nerve). By adding an interferon "boost," some of the cells that cause destruction are blocked and the disease is slowed down (modified) by about thirty percent. There are three choices of this drug type. A fourth option, a synthetic drug called Copaxone, acts differently, by not only blocking destructive cells, but creating more disease-fighting cells to reduce inflammation and lessen damage.

The material being attacked is called "myelin" and protects nerves much like the insulation that protects and insulates wires in an electrical system. I like this analogy of viewing the central nervous system like that of the wiring that runs through the walls of our homes.

I had helped do some rough electrical work once, and thought about how important it was to protect wiring from damage in order for the lights, fans, appliances and pumps to work properly. If there was a cut in the wiring or exposed wire at connection sites, the lights might not come on, would flicker intermittently, or would work well at first but then die out over time. I was to discover MS works much like this with damage to nerves instead of wire causing legs, hands, eyes, bladders and even brains to act like a damaged electrical system, sometimes undependable and sporadically functional. This destruction was referred to as "demyelination."

If a drug could slow this destruction down, I would take it! I finally acknowledged the reality of the disease and the fact that I needed help.

There are several kinds of MS. Relapsing-remitting is the most common kind in which symptoms come and go and a person may not be aware that anything destructive is happening, as in my case. Therefore, it is easy to miss, mistaking fatigue, forgetfulness and fleeting loss of strength as part of the human condition. Unfortunately, these are also symptoms of attacks in MS, compensated for at first by the body's amazing ability to regenerate itself, until a point of overload is reached (just like the electrical system). Symptoms are then obvious but damage cannot be reversed. Chronic progressive MS is less common, when the person experiences a steady, often rapid decline in ability. Secondary progressive MS is the type that follows a period of relapsing-remitting (anywhere from 10 to 20 years) and often changes to a slowed decline with less disease activity. A benign type is the least invasive form. I read versions of this general classification with warnings that MS acts differently for each person and is unpredictable in its course.

Disease-modifying drugs work only with relapsing-remitting MS, which is the type I was diagnosed with. Because I felt well except for chronic tiredness, I did not pursue any treatment for three years following my diagnosis. During this period, damage was likely occurring that could have been prevented.

I read about betas, alphas and gammas and was soon lost in a sea of medical terminology that was intimidating. I made a list to compare choices and summarize the information. It calmed my reeling brain.

DRUG CHOICES FOR RELAPSING-REMITTING MS
(as of 2001)
1. Avonex - 1996, (interferon beta-1a) - once per week/intramuscular injection
2. Rebif – 1998, (interferon beta-1a) – 3 times per week/subcutaneous injection
3. Betaseron – 1993, (interferon beta 1b) – every

other day / subcutaneous injection
4.   Copaxone – 1996, (glatiramer acetate) – every day / subcutaneous injection.

This list is already outdated because a fifth disease-modifying drug, Tysabri, was added in 2005.

Each of the interferons, (Avonex, Rebif, Betaseron), have flu-like side effects, ranging from mild to moderate, which normally subside over time as the body adjusts. The glatiramer acetate (Copaxone) has common injection-site reactions and possible chest pain. Mild site reactions are also common with interferons. *Subcutaneous* means a poke just below the surface of the skin and *intramuscular* is a deeper injection into the muscle.

I deliberated for a few days, read the details of each treatment and decided that an interferon was the best choice for me. Armed with information, I was impatient to start. It was almost five months before I could begin, due to the lengthy approval process.

~~~~~~

June was a challenging month. Teachers and students alike were weary of the school routine and ready for a break. The girls and I were excited about our summer plans for travelling and freedom from routine. Rachel was going to summer camp for a month in Vernon, British Columbia, through Army Cadets. We decided to paint the attic section of her bedroom before the trip. I bought supplies and Rachel picked out paint so we could start any time after school finished. I warned her it would be a lot of work, especially with the four-foot ceiling and limited room to move and stretch, but she was determined to give the room a makeover after the candle incident months before.

The last day of school finally came, and I stepped in the back door with relief, spilling books, gifts and bags across the table with a loud thunk.

"Yippee, two months off!" Becky danced around the kitchen as I sat down thankfully. The frenzied pace of field trips, special events, exams and farewells had worn me out. My job took a lot of energy.

Rachel walked in the door. "Hi. Do you think we could paint tomorrow?" Rachel had finished exams and classes almost a week ago and was keen to tackle the project.

"I really need a day to sleep in and get some chores done. How about the day after tomorrow? That would give you time to clear out the room."

"Okay, Mom, I'll do that. I can probably move most of the stuff myself."

"Be careful on the stairs." I had finally glued down carpet treads to make it less slippery. One of Becky's friends had slid down the last six steps and hurt her tailbone and it had scared me into action. She kept assuring me she was fine and I thanked God she was. I made it a priority, even though it felt like a never-ending list of things to take care of.

Sleeping in was heaven. I woke up to birds singing and a cat meowing at my door. I had the best job in the world, with two months off each year to rest and recover from busy full days that were beginning to wear me down. I worked in the garden, went grocery shopping and grilled steak on the barbeque.

We did not rush into painting the following day but began in a leisurely fashion after lunch. The "scritch" of sandpaper created a hot, dusty room, and we were soon sweating profusely. I wiped my forehead.

"Fun, eh? And we've barely begun. The painting will be the easy part!" The work was bringing back memories of past painting projects that sucked energy out of me.

"It'll be worth it though, Mom. I can't wait to see the new colour on the wall. Yellow will really brighten up the room." Rachel stopped sanding to gulp from her water bottle.

"What's that noise?" I stopped and listened closely. "You know, it sounds like a chain saw." My jaw dropped. "It can't be the neighbour here to cut down the trees. No one called. You keep working - I'll go and check."

I stepped out the front door to find a man running a chainsaw on our front lawn, and saw a large dump truck with my neighbour's company name, Radcliff Trucking, across the driver's door. Two more men were pulling chains, ropes and equipment from the truck. I rushed to put on my shoes.

My neighbour pulled up in his pick-up truck, stopped and rolled the window down, tipping his hat towards me.

"Let me know which trees you want cut. We'll start with that big one closest to my property." The whine of the machine drowned out anything more he had to say and he backed his truck up out of the way. I was stunned. There was no time to think, but I knew I did not want all the trees cut down.

I limped across the street to get a better view, and my neighbours joined me to survey the scene.

"Gosh, I didn't have any notice on this, so I'm feeling unprepared. On top of that, I'm in the middle of a painting project with Rachel, so the timing is rotten. But they're here, so I guess I had better figure out what I want." I tried to keep my frustration in check so I could think objectively.

"Well, Kathy, it's your property so don't let them do

158

anything you might regret. It's really unfortunate how they just showed up out of the blue." Another neighbour had joined us - a retiree who kept a close eye on things.

The first tree came down in thirds, from the top down, and the last section dropped with a loud "thwack" onto the sidewalk and front lawn. People drove by and slowed down to survey the scene; two vehicles turned around. I stepped in the front door as two men with chainsaws began cutting off branches and the dump truck pulled up adjacent to the house. They piled branches in the box.

"Hey, Rach," I hollered from the bottom of the stairs, "they're here to cut down the trees. Can you manage on your own for a while?" What choice did she have? I felt pulled in two directions.

"I'll come in when I get things sorted out."

"Go ahead, Mom. I'm fine."

I went outside and found my neighbour. "You can tell them to cut down the smaller tree beside the driveway." I looked at the foot-high stump beside the hedge from the first cut and glanced up at the power wires along the road. It was a dangerous job.

"What?"

"Cut down the tree beside the drive way," I yelled. He nodded.

"Cut them all down!" he yelled back, and I shook my head and mouthed the word **"NO."** I turned and hurried to move my SUV out of the driveway, parking several houses away. A small crowd gathered on the opposite side of the street and I joined them.

"Your leg's bothering you, isn't it, Kathy?" a kindly neighbour asked from where she stood leaning on a rake.

"Yes, I was trying to help Rachel paint her room when

these guys showed up, so it's created some stress." The faller was already up the next large tree that bordered my property. I looked for Dennis. He was nowhere in sight, and a "whirrrr" from the chain saw filled the air as the next tree top fell with a splintering crash.

"Do you want that tree cut down, Kathy? Weren't you thinking of every other tree?" I watched the scene helplessly.

"I'm really torn between having more light and keeping the trees. I think this will make my living room brighter." Maybe I should let them take all the trees. The manpower and equipment were here and it wasn't costing me any money. I stood watching, speechless, as the next treetop came tumbling down and almost landed in the back of a pick-up truck that had slowed to peek up at the faller. The woman sped up quickly as she heard the crack of a tree splitting, and the treetop hit the pavement, narrowly missing her truck.

The narrow escape spurred me into action. Dennis was behind the wheel of the dump truck parked in his driveway, waiting for the crew to buck up another load of branches that would be hauled to the dump.

"Hey, Dennis," I yelled, "that's enough cutting. There are only two trees left and that's plenty of light for us." He nodded and I watched his hunched figure in conversation with the crew leader. He seemed satisfied and I stood on guard until I was sure no more trees were going to be cut and the small group that had gathered dispersed. Rachel needed me now. Becky had gone down the street to play with her friend.

"Wow, Rachel, look at the work you've done," I commented when I dragged myself upstairs. "I see you've done more repairs. That's really going to make a difference."

"I think we can start painting." She stared at the piece

160

of drywall we had sealed up from the spooky part of the attic. "I'll start here and work my way over to the stairs."

"I'll follow you with the brush and do the edges." At least I could sit while doing this.

"So, Rachel, you should see the front yard. They took out four of the six trees, and it looks empty. Plus, I'm exhausted." My voice broke and a few tears slipped out.

"Don't worry, Mom. We'll get used to it and it should be a lot brighter. Remember all the times you wished it wasn't so dark?" Rachel moved back from the wall she had finished. "Speaking of bright, look at this! I love it." The yellow was brilliant as the late afternoon sun swung round and poured into the room. We finished before dark. The room smelled like fresh paint and glowed in the setting sun.

The following morning we slept in late and I stopped in the threshold of my doorway that faced the front yard. The missing trees left a huge void filled with telephone wires, a thick, creosoted pole, roadway and our neighbour's small, red brick house. His meticulously kept lawns and gardens were in stark contrast to the patchy brown lawn that was my own. Once again, my eyes stung. It was only some silly trees, I told myself. I had grown used to their scraggly protection and I was unprepared for the rapid change. I did grow to appreciate the added sunlight, however, and eventually filled the space with some lilac bushes and added another flower garden under Rachel's bedroom window.

Becky and I travelled to the lush Okanagan Valley of British Columbia two weeks later and spent a weekend in Vernon visiting Rachel, who was at cadet camp until August. We met Kelly-Leigh, her sister and niece and made an adventure of travelling down to Vancouver, stopping to camp in the mountains that bordered the Fraser Valley near Hope, making last minute plans to see a "Guess Who" concert before Kelly-Leigh's veterinary conference began. It was a whirlwind of fun and we ended up downtown in a hotel adjacent to the ocean and Stanley Park. I walked several blocks without any problem, encouraged by a boost of energy and a sense of well-being. The tree-cutting incident seemed long, long ago.

The weather was glorious, not too hot but sunny and bright and we spent the week visiting family, friends and going out in the evenings with Kelly-Leigh. The trip home, about 1000 kilometres through several mountains ranges, was pleasant except for the last few hours when we were travel weary. I found the drive soothing, a time to think, reflect and soak in magnificent scenery. Becky fell asleep several times, which made it easier to continue driving and before I knew it we were in Mount Robson Provincial Park, less than two hours from home. We began stopping more often, played silly word games and "I spy" as we cruised along, and sang "The Song That Never Ends" at the top of our lungs.

Becky had ten days at home before she went to spend time with her Dad and after she was gone, I began preparing in earnest for a camping trip with my cousin in an arid lake region of the BC Okanagan on Shuswap Lake. It was renowned for its clean, warm water, boating, fishing and recreation. Rachel lent me her tent, and after organizing all the supplies, I estimated there was enough room left to pack my mountain bike. There were some biking trails near our campground along the Adams River, famous for its fall salmon runs, and I intended to ride them if possible. I could bike much further than I could walk and felt a great sense of accomplishment when I rode.

I planned to have a friend come in and feed the cat while I was gone, but never had to make the arrangements. Our nocturnal cat disappeared one evening, never to return. I walked the neighbourhood several times and biked round, calling his name, certain he would appear. On the third day, after calling the SPCA and the Animal Pound, I made some posters and taped them to mailboxes around the neighbourhood.

MISSING - A white and brown 3-year-old male **CAT**, since Monday, July 29. He didn't come home, and he's in big trouble. PLEASE CALL 865-2618

Using our coloured printer, I added a picture and printed out half a dozen copies. My computer skills were improving. I thought about the cat's loyal companionship. The girls would be very upset if he did not come home. He was a big, sixteen-pound male, tough and skilled in the outdoors. I went camping a week later without our cat reappearing.

Camping was wonderful. It was restful and relaxing, and Barb and I were becoming friends, something we had never had a chance to do before. The water was warm and I swam around the perimeter of the roped off area almost everyday, doing plenty of reading, sleeping, sun tanning and enjoying delicious food. The beach was gravelly and I vowed to buy some "water shoes" for next time because the rocks dug into my feet. Biking was invigorating as the trail dipped and curved through the trees, narrow, but not difficult to navigate. A cooling breeze off the water and shade from the dense forest kept me from over-heating.

As Barb and I lay on the beach in the shade, Bernadette's words came back to me. "Your writing is wonderful, Kathy. The poems are filled with emotion and meaning. They touch my heart. Keep on writing." I wrote a poem for my good friend, who was on a journey of her own, in a worldly adventure with her family to the Dominican Republic. Her dream of teaching in another country was unfolding because she had accepted a one-year posting to teach in a tropical paradise. I valued her friendship and knew we would stay in touch. Our paths kept crossing in unexpected ways.

My thoughts shifted deep into the past as my eyes closed and my body became fluid like the water beside me.

~~~~~~

I could feel Dave's intense pleasure in my appearance as his focus shifted to the project he had put his heart and soul into. Our house. I had been away working while he had spent the summer building and framing the place of his imagination, which he had built many times over in his dreams. Every detail had been thought out, carefully crafted and ingeniously constructed with care, precision, and an engineer's mind.

"Come up here," he beckoned. "It's an interesting perspective that you've got to see." He held out his hand and I scrambled up the truss. Dave disappeared high above. He clambered around on the two by fours like a monkey, confident in his skill.

"This is really cool," I lied, as I concentrated, shinnying across the narrow board. My knuckles turned white as I gripped the wood, and my eyes travelled down, down to the pit below me that was filled with boulders, gravel and sand that sandwiched the large corrugated tubes where warm air would be pumped to heat the floor. A slab of concrete would be poured over the layers.

"Hey, Dave," called Steven, our young neighbour and Dave's helper for the summer. "Come look at this." I was relieved to have Dave's attention drawn away from me. I

trembled at the void of space that loomed above and below. I shook myself. Since when had I been afraid of heights? What was wrong with me? Hadn't I clambered up a steep concrete roof only two years previously at firefighting training school? A steel ladder, bulky fire-fighting gear, heavy breathing apparatus and slippery boots had not stopped me. Maybe I had been too busy concentrating on the simulated fire to be scared of heights. In a panic, I had struggled to hook up my breathing apparatus as smoke poured into the building, but it was not the paralyzing fear that choked me now.

I saw Steven at the top level in the corner of the roof, and I forced myself to join him as Dave scurried across the narrow boards like a squirrel, perfectly at home, with a work apron tied loosely at his waist and a pencil tucked behind one ear.

"How can you be so confident way up here?"

He laughed. "I don't know. It feels comfortable to me, kind of like a second skin. Why don't you come over here?"

"No thanks, this is good for me. You go ahead and do what ever it is you were going to." I looked three floors down into the basement, and my head began to spin as nausea threatened to overwhelm me. I grabbed a corner board to steady myself. Frozen, I crouched motionless, pretending to admire the view. My hands gripped the boards as I lowered myself back to a partially completed floor and took a deep, calming breath.

"Let's hammer some flooring down," suggested Dave as he joined me. Steven made it a trio and soon the satisfying tink of nails sinking into solid wood rang out.

"This isn't so bad." I was appreciating a firm floor beneath my feet.

"This floor will never squeak given the number of nails we've pounded into it. Just wait until the bigger nails need to be hammered from underneath the roof. Now that will be hard work." When the time came, I was barely able to manage the feat, twisting my neck and back into the most awkward positions attempting to get enough weight behind the monster *nails. My hands had just recovered from several weeks of "rock throwing," picking up and pitching boulder-sized rocks down the giant culverts into the basement area. Dave could barely open his hands at the end of each day. I felt like a woman of Kleenex beside a man of steel.*

~~~~~~

The sun had moved across the sky and the weeping willow no longer provided the shade that had been so pleasant. I opened my eyes to see Barb had moved to a new shady spot, her big straw hat bent towards the book she held. As I dipped into the cooling water, a powerboat cruising beyond the divider created large waves that rolled, dipped, crashed and began their rhythm all over again, becoming gentle ripples by the time they reached shore. It was so peaceful here.

When Becky and I met in Hinton, I broke the news about our missing cat.

"But, Mom, I never got to say good-bye. I love Snowy." She began to cry. I cried too, re-opening the wound that had barely healed from my own sense of loss.

"I'm so sorry, Beck. There's a small chance we'll get him back, but I don't want you to get your hopes up." In fact he did not return and we spent the last weeks of the summer sad in the knowledge that we had lost our cat. We still had to get organized for the school year and finish odd jobs. I painted part of the white wooden fence, dug another small garden and rode my bike with Becky. We tackled a longer-than-usual ride to the "Hill" district, and even though we were both very tired afterwards, I was proud of our accomplishment. I sat for a long time before I had the strength to get up.

TEN

"O, say can you see,
by the dawn's early light..."
~American Anthem ~

September 11, 2001. I will never forget the sense of horror and shock we felt in our families, workplace and the community as the day unfolded and we learned about the terrorist attacks in the United States. I walked home quickly on my lunch break and sat stiffly in front of the television as the news grew more unreal. So many innocent people had died a terrifying death. So many more people had lost loved ones, or worse, did not have any confirmation one way or another. I prayed for the people affected by the horrific, senseless tragedy. How could an event like this happen in a civilized society? My mind reeled with confusion, always looking first for the good in mankind. There was none here on this judgment day.

Bernadette was teaching in Santo Domingo, Dominican Republic when this event rocked the world and she emailed me.

"I just want to come home. The world doesn't feel safe anymore, and we're going crazy adjusting to a very different culture than ours, sweating everyday in the blasting heat, and living in cramped quarters with crazy

Dominicans screaming all around us."

Not only were she and her family dealing with culture shock, but adding terrorist shock from the World Trade Center attacks increased their sensory and visual overload to the breaking point. They were far from their comfort zone.

I communicated my empathy and a thought grew as we corresponded. "If your friend Lewis is coming to see you, maybe Becky and I will come and visit while you're there. It would be a big adventure!"

"We would like that, Kathy. Maybe next spring would work. I'll check the dates I'm off. The boys would love the company." Becky and Ben were close to the same age.

In my Bible study group, through our church, we had finished a study on baptism. Now that I understood the connection between God, Jesus and the Holy Spirit, I was considering the next step. The Trinity was an unknown to me, incomplete in my mind and spirit, but now that I understood the relationship, the act of faith would help me move forward. I wanted clear direction for my life through that faith.

I did not know at the time it would be so hard to be "in the world, but not of the world." The pressures in our society to be a unique individual do not match Christian values to conform and follow, but I learned we can still use our talents and individual "gifts" to help others and better the world. A huge weight lifted from my shoulders to be the "hero."

Was happiness the ultimate goal or a myth spun by books, fairytales and modern man? Was chasing an elusive "feeling" unrealistic and fruitless? I did not expect everything that happened to bring me constant happiness. I saw that feelings ebb and flow and are fragile. I was starting to recognize that trials and suffering are part of our time on earth for everyone, and that they form and shape us. It was necessary to trust, letting go of control and understanding life is not just a series of random events.

My thinking was shifting from what the world tells us to expect to what God tells us. It helped me understand that multiple sclerosis was part of my life for a reason and that I didn't have to like it, but I needed to learn to live, cope and change with it.

At the end of August, our cat had been gone for over a month so we started visiting the local SPCA.

"Mom, can we go to the SPCA tonight to see the animals? Maybe we could walk a dog."

"Sure, let's ride our bikes. I can't promise to walk a dog, but we'll see." I knew Becky wanted a dog, but it was too big a commitment for me. Cats were a better choice for us. I was considering adopting another cat, but hesitated to share my thoughts with Becky, whose enthusiasm was contagious and threatened to cloud my judgment. No kittens, no dogs. She would not understand, but I knew what I could handle.

It was cool and cloudy when we arrived shortly after a volunteer unlocked the door in the early evening. The long daylight hours were slowly fading in the last bit of summer glory and in a few short months, darkness would be upon us at this time, bikes would be stored away, and nature would lie dormant in the endless cycle of rest and renewal.

We leaned our bikes up against a concrete wall. A single vehicle was parked outside the Shelter and dogs began barking as soon as we approached.

"Whoof, whoof, rar, rar, rar, rar, ahrooooo..." went the cacophony of greetings as we passed by the cages. My bicycle helmet barely muted the deafening sound of dogs in cages, man's best friend confined and lonely for human company.

"Oh, Mom, look at this dog!" Becky hollered above the din.

"Let's go inside and see the cats first," I yelled back. We stepped inside the door and shut it rapidly.

"Look at the kittens! They're so cute." We stood admiring the older kittens and heard a loud bark behind another closed door.

The door opened and two large mixed-breed dogs came bounding into the small office area and sniffed all over Becky. I was next, and the taller dog stuck his nose in my crotch as I pushed him away, retreating to the cat room where I was less likely to be knocked over and licked to death. Becky followed me and we looked into the larger cage where a tabby sat calmly observing us.

"Ohhhh, that cat is sweet, Mom. Can we go in the cage and hold it, please, please?"

"Hang on, I'll ask." I went to find the volunteer, who was busy in the large warehouse-style room cleaning empty dog cages.

"Yes, just make sure the cat or cats go back in the same cage they came out of before you open a different one."

"Thanks."

Becky and I went inside the cage and visited with the quiet tabby, which seemed very gentle and calm. Big almond-shaped green eyes blinked up at me. We spent some time visiting with all the cats except the mama who was ready to give birth. The information sheet on the tabby said it was a ten-month old female, "Missy," spayed and with her shots up-to-date.

We walked a smaller dog to the end of the dusty road and back, and Becky was satisfied. The dog pulled hard on the leash and barked considerably, so it was a relief to hand him over. When we returned home and stored our bikes in the shed, I pulled the cat carrier off a shelf and dusted cobwebs and grime away. Becky jumped up and down.

"Are we gonna bring home the cat we both liked so much? I love you, Mom." She could barely contain her excitement as we prepared to go and collect the cat.

"She's perfect for us, Becky. Not a little kitten, but not quite grown up yet, either. I loved her personality, calm and sweet. She purred so easily when I picked her up."

So Missy's life began with us, and she is still with us today, a beautiful mild-mannered creature who is loyal, loving and independent.

~~~~~~

The teacher-aide course I had taken gave me a fresh perspective in the classroom and a few new ideas to help kids struggling in reading and math. Melissa was in grade five. The difference between Melissa and her peers was growing as rapidly as she was, and I was job sharing with a new teacher aide since Shirley had been reassigned to a different student. Shirley found the job too physically demanding and needed a change. I was reaching that point myself but not ready to admit it.

Melissa needed more coaxing, lifting, support and direction than ever before. She had entered puberty, a year older than most children in her class, and her mood swings were hard to deal with on some days. I was finding the swimming routine particularly tiring, even though she had a wonderful, patient instructor who took her in the water.

Debilitating headaches plagued me that fall, some of which caused me to stumble and see double, and I missed the odd day of work because of it. Was MS going to attack my sight, too?

At home, our furnace finally broke down. I arranged to have it replaced with a new, efficient one, and could not wait to have a little more heat and less rattling. Winter usually began around Halloween, with cold temperatures and big snowfalls, but we were lucky to have the new system in place just in time.

The old furnace and ducting were strewn across the lawn when I arrived home from work, and the man in charge was cursing and swearing as they continued to throw material out of the back door. I wanted a second heat vent in the chilly kitchen hooked up, which required plenty of extra crawling around in a dusty tight space and elicited more bad language. It cost a fortune but that seemed to be the nature of repairing an older home.

I tried to interest my kids. "Listen, girls, it's so much quieter except when it first starts up. It sounds a bit like a jet engine." Becky was watching television.

"U-huh."

"Don't you think it's a lot warmer?" I wanted feedback.

"Yeah, I guess so." I attempted to interest my fifteen-year-old, who was in the bathroom doing laundry.

"Hey, Rachel, what d'you think about our new furnace? Nice and warm, huh?" The bathroom did not even have a heat vent because it sat above the crawl space, directly above the furnace.

"It's quieter, Mom. What's for dinner?" Furnaces were obviously not a hot kid topic, but I was grateful to have a new one!

~~~~~~

In keeping with tradition, snow arrived at Halloween. As I drove across the icy, snowy logging road to Robb to take Becky to her Dad, traffic was light and I put the vehicle in four-wheel drive on the slippery stretches. On the return trip, I was satisfied with the grip the tires seemed to have and drove without engaging the four-by-four. My thoughts drifted to the trip to Edmonton I was making with a fellow teacher assistant on Thursday to learn more about a touch-screen computer program the school had purchased. Melissa liked computers but was unable to manipulate the mouse correctly or understand the correlation between mouse, keyboard and screen.

The road straightened out and I automatically increased my speed. It felt too fast, even though I was under the speed limit, so I applied the brakes and in an instant the vehicle slid off the road and flipped over. I sat for a minute in stunned disbelief.

I took a deep breath, then another. How could I be so calm? This was my second accident on the same road and my brain refused to register the bizarre coincidence. The seatbelt was jammed and kept me locked into place, which forced me to stop and look around. The normal order of the world had been reversed, and my sense of spatial connection was disrupted like the misfiring neurons of multiple sclerosis.

My eyes surveyed the dim interior and came to rest on the spare tire that was shoved up against the smoked glass of the rear driver's side. I did not see any broken glass or dented metal. I shivered. That loose tire was a potential missile that I had known about but ignored. The danger stared me in the face as I continued to breathe.

The horn still worked and I pushed hard. "Honk, honk, hoooonk." There had been few vehicles on the road, but it was getting dark and most workers had finished their shift and gone home. I pressed the horn again and again. The whirring of an engine reached my altered auditory sense and I suddenly realized the sound was my own truck. I turned the engine off. Dead silence.

Within a couple of minutes I heard a vehicle stop and a voice reached my ears.

"You okay, lady?"

"I think so. If I unbuckle the seatbelt, will I drop very far?" I was worried about my shifting weight causing the vehicle to move.

"No, it should be all right. The seatbelt's jammed so I'll use my knife to cut it." In a few seconds, I was free and my feet were on the ground. Strong hands helped me out and I stood for a minute looking at the flipped SUV. In the fading light, it appeared undamaged. It had been cushioned by the soft snow that held it in place.

"You're sure you're okay?" I rubbed my arms and shivered.

"Not a scratch. It's a miracle." We recovered my purse, and zombie-like, I followed my rescuer to a warm truck.

"Pretty slippery out tonight. Do you live in Hinton?"

"Yes. I took my daughter to Robb and was returning home to Hinton. That ice really caught me by surprise. One second I was driving, and 'boom', the next second I was in the ditch."

"That's how it happens sometimes. I'll take you home if you want." We made the remainder of the trip in silence.

"Thanks so much. I appreciate it," I said as I stepped into my driveway.

"Glad I could help, good luck."

The door was unlocked and lights were on, and I went to find Rachel.

"You'll never believe what happened. I had another car accident, a roll over, so we don't have any wheels right now." I tried to wish the accident away.

"You mean you can't drive me up to Kim's? Maaaahmom!" Rachel stormed out, slamming the door

174

behind her. I put my head down on the table and began to cry. She had not even asked me if I was okay. I cried and cried.

"Ding-dong." The doorbell rang but I ignored it. Trick or treaters were starting to arrive so I got up, turned out the lights and grabbed the phone. I will call Kristin. She was a wonderful listener and prayed aloud at our Bible study meetings with insight, caring and compassion. She arrived a few minutes later and I flipped the lights back on. I sat on the bench by the back door as Kristin stood very still listening to my story. As I relived the accident, shaking overtook my body. Kristin sat down, put her arm around me, and began to pray. She prayed through my tears, shaking, the doorbell ringing and voices outside, wondrously transforming Biblical teaching into words that brought me comfort and understanding, words that brought meaning to my life that I could relate to; gradually the shaking subsided. Conviction poured through me.

"I want to be baptized! As soon as possible – do you think Daren could do it this Sunday?" For a minute, I forgot about the accident.

We talked a little more, and Kristin left. I felt much better.

I phoned to let the school know I would not be in the next day, and rode with the tow truck driver to recover the vehicle. When we rounded the corner where the truck sat, we exclaimed aloud at the same time.

"Wow!" The truck was nothing like what I remembered or described to him.

"It's much further off the road than I expected. What a huge right-of-way. Good thing I have a really long cable winch, probably have to use a tree up there," he said, pointing to the line of bush that began past the clearing. The SUV was twenty feet off the road.

It took a long time to right the vehicle and winch it slowly across the snow. Once all four wheels were touching the ground, we could see the roof had absorbed the impact. The large crease in the metal was obvious and as it moved towards us, a dent in the hood became visible. Yikes, it really was amazing I was unhurt. I guess God still wanted me around and I was so grateful.

There was no point in dwelling on something out of my control and after getting organized with a courtesy car from the auto-body shop, making a statement at the police station, and having a doctor confirm I was fine, I decided to carry on with my plans to travel to Edmonton the following day. Rachel did not say much, but I thought she was a bit freaked out by my bad driving record. I tried not to be. There were too many other things to think about, like a new vehicle to replace the second write-off in five years.

I was very sad to lose the SUV. It was ideal for our lifestyle, living in snow-bound West Central Alberta. It made sense to replace it with something similar so within two days I had just the vehicle picked out at a dealership only a few blocks from our house. It was a simple transition, and the insurance payout covered the cost - more blessings from heaven. I had lived the importance of having proper insurance twice.

It was dark when we travelled to Edmonton for the touch-screen computer course the next morning and dark again when we returned. It had been a long day but a good way for me to cope with the events of the past forty-eight hours. I went to bed early for a long, dreamless sleep. I found the best way to manage most kinds of stress was to get busy and carry on whenever possible.

The staffroom was a flurry of activity when I entered

on Friday morning for my coffee break and I plunked down in a chair, eyeing the tempting treats on the table.

"We heard about the accident, Kathy. Glad you're okay."

"Thanks, it was a bit of a shock. " I scooped up a gooey brownie.

"Did your car have a lot of damage?"

"It didn't seem like it at first, but it doesn't take much with older vehicles to add up to a write-off. My SUV was ten years old." I got up and poured a coffee, and when the bell rang, I remembered to check my mailbox before leaving. There was a yellow note stuffed in the cubbyhole.

"Kathy, call hospital reception at 865-3581." I phoned the number.

"Hi, Kathy, yes we have an appointment date for the MS nurse to meet with you. She'll come to your house, if that works. You need to have your medication ready. It's on Tuesday evening, at seven o'clock."

"Thanks." I scribbled the information down and hurried upstairs.

I already had the box of three syringes in my fridge at home and the company that made the interferon had sent me a starter kit with an injector, alcohol swabs, a diary, and a "how-to" video. I was nervous, but excited about taking a pro-active approach to managing this contrary disease, which went up and down like a yo-yo. At the top of the spin I felt good, but as the string unwound and the yo-yo descended, I felt weak and spun out of control. This was the relapsing (feeling bad), remitting (feeling good) pattern that I had read so much about.

The local MS Society had sent me an envelope full of booklets, brochures, and information that I dug into, wondering why I had waited so long to take this seriously. I pretended to myself that everything was fine, when indeed it was not. It was truly a disease of denial. I read the booklet on *"Ten Tips for People Living With MS"* twice, and almost used it like a mantra:

"Be Educated, Listen to Your Body, You are the Same Person as You Were, Stay Healthy, Manage Your Mood, Involve Your Family, Develop a Support Network, Plan for the Future, Stay Positive, Stand Up For Yourself."

I highlighted something that was intuitive and practical.

"A painter who loses his sight may become a sculptor. Learn to cope with the curveballs that life throws. Change what you can. Accept what you must. Live your life as richly as you did before."

The nurse sat in the cold kitchen with me as we talked. She suggested I take acetaminophen fifteen minutes before the injection, and take a single syringe out of the fridge about the same time to take the chill out of the clear liquid that was pre-measured in the syringe.

"Let's start with your thigh, using inner fatty tissue." I pulled up my stretchy sweat pants and patted a damp alcohol swab on the injection site. The nurse simulated how to load the injector, and then I did it myself with the syringe.

"The beauty of this system is that you don't have to put the needle in. The injector does it for you, after you place it lightly over the skin, and then push the button. Voila, it's done!" I waited a minute, and then pushed the button, holding my breath. Nothing happened.

"It's not working! What am I doing wrong?"

"It might be a bit stiff since it's new, try pressing a little harder."

"Zing." I felt a light pinch and lifted the injector off my thigh. A tiny pool of blood rose to the surface and we blotted it with paper towel. Within a few seconds, it had stopped bleeding.

"I guess that wasn't so bad."

"You might find the site turns red and burns a bit, but it doesn't usually last more than a few days." The nurse started to put on her coat. "If you have any questions, or you'd like me to come over again, just call." She smiled encouragingly, collected her things, and was gone.

That was it. The kids and I went to bed early, and I only woke once in the night for my usual trip to the bathroom. The following morning I had almost forgotten about "disease modifying therapy."

Two nights later, I injected myself without too much difficulty, but tossed and turned a bit in the night and woke feeling slightly warm. I took the suggested ibuprofen and went to work. Most nights I slept through and adjusted to the routine slowly, making mistakes like dropping the injector on the floor and losing a syringe full of medication, missing the target (like my bum: much harder to see than my thighs) and hesitating before self-inflicting a pinch. Sometimes the injections hurt. Sometimes I felt nothing. The doctor explained this would continue to happen, given the random nature of the injection sites and the fact that what was underneath the skin varied from muscle fibres to blood vessels, etc. There was no science to this method. The needle piercing the skin only went in about a quarter of an inch. I put the used needles in a plastic container marked "Bio-hazardous Material" and took it to the pharmacy when it was full.

It was time to meet the psychologist again. My

employer provided an excellent extended health care program that included this service. I knew it was important to talk to an objective person that could help me cope with what felt like a heavy weight at times - a full-time job, two children to feed and provide a home for, and a disease that was sneaking in like a thief in the night, robbing me of precious energy and physical ability. Some were chosen circumstances, others not. We wrestled through questions that threatened to overwhelm me and the psychologist helped me see I had choices and even opportunity.

For me, the baptism that followed a month later was a joy and an honour. It was funny, too, because I did not have a church background, but many seeds had been planted along the way that I was not even aware of. In a brief year, I had learned enough to know with certainty I wanted to make this commitment. I had never seen a baptism and had vague recollections of my close friend Helene's account of hers and her husband's baptism in the same church over ten years before. She had been nervous about the dunking (a small, warm tank is provided). I was nervous about descending a few stairs into the water because stairs were becoming difficult to navigate without a handrail. I was also excited.

Did I have doubts? Of course. Many things in the Bible I did not fully understand or was even aware of, but for me the decision was akin to marriage or having a baby or nurturing a deep friendship. It was all about relationships and I was entering into a personal relationship with God. The Bible was now my reference point to deal with life.

"What do we do if there's something we don't agree with in the Bible?" I asked one day in our small group. My question was answered with a question.

"What do you do if there's a rule or law you don't

agree with?" I paused in thought.

"Hmmm, I guess I follow it anyway or maybe I break it, get caught, and get punished. Like a speeding ticket." Everyone laughed.

"You know, we often do things we don't feel like doing, and the Bible is no different. It's all about trust and letting go of controlling everything."

I thought about the words to a song we sang in church. "It's all about you, Jesus ... It's not about me, as if you should do things my way ...You alone are God ... and I surrender to your ways." I was so weary of trying to do it all myself, and God knew exactly what I needed, even if it was a car accident or a chronic disease, or two beautiful daughters or a wonderful job. It was all there, in the "Book of Life."

~~~~~~

Another Christmas was upon us, and I welcomed the two-week break from work. Kelly-Leigh wanted us to meet her in Banff to go downhill skiing, so my daughters and I planned to meet her the day after New Year's.

It would be my first trip away from home with the new medication routine. I was anxious to see if I could still manage a few "bunny" runs down the mountain, and my kids were looking forward to another adventure with their adopted aunt. Kelly-Leigh referred to Rachel and Becky as her "godchildren" and took her commitment seriously, sincerely and happily. We were so blessed to have someone who cared so much about our well-being. Almost effortlessly, she entered our lives with more caring and support than I had felt in years. She would unexpectedly put money into my bank account, often at times when I wondered how I would afford the next grocery shopping. I told her she was my guardian angel, thanking God in my prayers for such a wonderful friend.

When the newly acquired SUV broke down a few days before we were scheduled to drive to Banff, I had mixed feelings. I was dreading driving through the snow-covered mountains, but also did not want my dear friend to ski alone for the week. I was willing to make the trip to spend time with her and promote further bonding between her and the girls. Kristin called and I told her of my situation. The shop could not get the part in time for my vehicle to be repaired.

A few hours later, the phone rang again.

"Hi, Kathy. Daren and I would like to lend you our van so that you don't have to cancel your trip to Banff. He and Nicholas are cleaning it out right now."

"But that's your only vehicle! We'll be gone for five days, and you have a family of four to take care of." I was amazed they would trust me with their van. I had just had the accident two months before.

"Kathy, it's not a problem for us. We can walk everywhere, the church is close, and Daren's back is bothering him so he doesn't plan to go far. Please accept our offer."

"I'm overwhelmed, but yes, that would work beautifully." We discussed a few details and I went to tell my kids the news that the trip was still on.

It was a winter wonderland on the Icefields Parkway as we started out. The sun shone on the snow-covered hills, tree boughs glistened, drooping with the weight of soft white powder. The valleys that caught the sun's rays sparkled and danced. They were like skaters whirling around an outdoor ice rink. The road climbed, dropped, curved and straightened out into the open valleys by magnificent mountain peaks that rose up into an azure blue sky to dazzle even the most uninterested passenger. We followed the route through a narrow passage beside a frozen waterfall, where climbers blended into the rock as invisible as the Rocky Mountain big horn sheep we had passed earlier, until the eye caught movement and suddenly they stood out starkly.

We travelled a little further and the landscape opened into large windblown rocks devoid of trees. To the west, a glacier swept down the mountain where an unusual all-terrain vehicle with huge, knobby tires sat waiting to transport people into a timeless world of frozen ice. In the background, another glacier sat hanging above, tucked in the shadows, creating a classic circular shape that was feathered with wrinkles and large cracks. We pulled into a large, almost empty parking lot. Wind whipped the snow around creating little tornados and I quickly changed my mind about stopping.

We passed Parker's Ridge, an area that looked slightly familiar, and I recognized it as a place I had cross-country skied once many years before. The road snaked around the back of the mountain and descended in a tight circle onto a huge, flat plain of frozen water and rock. I massaged the tension in my neck with my left hand as the road straightened out. We had driven highway that was bare, windswept, a sea of dusty powder, hard-packed with snow, rough and bumpy, slippery and icy – always changing like a chameleon, keeping drivers alert and cautious.

Between Lake Louise and Banff, the highway became double lanes in both directions and drivers increased their speed just as a fine snow began to fall in the dusk. The van seemed to hang low to the ground and felt stable under my feet despite the slippery conditions, but I drew in a quick breath when we passed a car in the ditch. We could not get there soon enough.

Several miles later, another vehicle had spun around

and landed in the right-of-way between the traffic, doors were flung open and a woman was stumbling around in the snow carrying a small child, with several people following her. Cars had pulled over on the side of the road. Another vehicle hung in the ditch with a broken windshield and a large dent in the side door, seemingly abandoned. We heard a siren in the distance; people had stopped to help, so we continued.

I shivered. The scene haunted me and I fretted aloud.

"That was scary. Hope we get there soon. Will you girls watch for the Banff exit sign?"

"Can't, Mom. Becky's sleeping and I don't have my glasses on. When will we be there?"

"Soon, really soon, I think." Please God, keep us safe on this treacherous road. We passed another car in the ditch and a tow-truck driving the opposite way.

I relayed the story to my friend that evening while we warmed up during a lovely meal. The next morning, she offered to drive and I gratefully handed her the keys.

"The gondola is really long and gets us high into the mountain for the best skiing. There are a couple of chalets where we can have lunch." We stood in a long line-up to buy our tickets and my feet froze in my light-duty hiking boots. Maybe I could warm my feet up in the gondola. The temperature posted at the ticket booth was minus 15 degrees Celsius.

The girls were excited. "Are you going to ski with us, Mom?" Becky asked, and I nodded.

"Maybe you can come down an easier run with me first."

"But Mom, I go kind of fast," she warned.

"That's okay; you can stop and wait for me if you get really far ahead." The unheated gondola climbed and climbed, but all we could see was snow and trees as the clouds swallowed us. Even with insulated ski boots, my feet remained numb. They would warm up once I got moving.

I decided to attempt the first run by myself, a kind of test-run with no one else to keep up to, while Kelly-Leigh and the girls went off to find a more challenging route. I rode the chair to the top of an intermediate run. This was not a place for novice skiers; the hills were steep and the moguls were large. The wind was biting, my hands and feet were frozen, and visibility was poor. I dug my poles in, determined to prove to myself I could still ski.

There was no pleasure left in it. From top to bottom, the run was a torturous, gruelling marathon to my shocked system. Turning took all the strength in my legs. I crisscrossed the slopes and picked myself up again and yet again. All the determination in the world was not going to lead me down the mountain. It was survival and I choked back my fear.

It took an hour to get down a slope that would have taken me ten minutes in the past. I collapsed on a chair inside the chalet and did not move until Kelly-Leigh, Rachel and Becky showed up half an hour later. I told them briefly what had happened, and they brought me a steaming hot chocolate.

"If you go through that door and turn left, there's a fireplace where you could warm yourself," Kelly-Leigh said as they left. They promised to return for lunch, and I sat until my bladder forced me to move. My legs felt like wooden sticks, unbendable and not my own. I hobbled to the bathroom. I spent the rest of the day near the fireplace with a book, but my legs did not recover their usual strength. The lift operator slowed the gondola so that I could take small steps to get into it. If I needed any confirmation my skiing days were over, this was it. I was devastated. The nurturing I had found in nature had suddenly turned hostile.

The rest of the week was a bit of a blur. The supporting arm of my girlfriend led me to a fabulous meal of rack of lamb, and we relaxed in a warm, soothing hot tub and a pool fed by hot springs. The numbing cold of the outdoors hindered my recovery, and I limped about with dry eyes, jabbing the needle into my arm on the injection nights.

The five-hour trip home seemed long, uneventful and tiring. The road was dry and clear of snow. The girls complained and fought as we headed north but I tried to shut out the dissention. The clear blue sky and blazing sun compelled me to look beyond my troubled thoughts at the majestic peaks. I was now unable to climb those peaks and fought to accept my new limitations.

~~~~~~

January was a time of adjusting to routine, cocooning at home, and planning our trip to the Dominican Republic in March, during spring break. I applied for passports and an extra week off in order to have a couple of days of rest at each end of the ten-day trip. Rachel was not interested in coming and wanted to stay with her friends.

My legs slowly regained strength but I was careful to wear warm winter clothing, especially boots, whenever I was outdoors and this seemed to help. I started driving to work in the mornings too, even though it was only three blocks away. I needed to conserve my energy for work, shopping, errands and caring for my kids and home. When I expressed guilt to my friends over the anti-environmental choice I was making, they empathized with me by saying I could easily replace my car but not my legs. Once again, it was necessary to adapt to the disease in order to carry on.

It was hard to tell whether the interferon was working because I did not feel any different. In fact, maybe I was a tiny bit stiffer, but at least had worked through the titration of the drug without any major side effects. I had to trust it was slowing demyelination even if I could not tell.

I had had a poem published in an anthology of verse written by people of all different ages and backgrounds, including children. I marked several pages in the book for Becky, keeping in mind the annual poetry recital contest at school. Each student needed to memorize and recite a poem at his or her grade level. Most students picked from a selection of half a dozen poems given to them by their teacher.

"Do you like any of the poems you brought home, Becky? Why don't you pick one to recite?"

"I like these two, but lots of kids are doing them." As I read the poems, she recited the first one from memory.

"Wow, that was very good. I liked your actions. This poetry book I have has a few kids' poems you could look at if you want to try something different." She disappeared with the heavy book and returned a few minutes later.

"I like this one." She pointed to a poem titled "Homework," written by a child her age, and started to recite. "Homework oh homework, you're a pain in the neck … you fill up my backpack till nothing will fit." By the time Becky finished we were both laughing hard, and she repeated it several times, experimenting with different actions as she went along.

"It's a funny poem, Becky, and it suits you!"

"Would I be able to do it for the contest?"

"I don't see why not, but I'll check tomorrow at school and get you a photocopy." To my amazement, she won first place and had the intimidating task of reciting it in front of an audience of four hundred school-aged kids, their teachers, and a few parents. I was very proud of her.

I worried about my oldest daughter's dislike of school. She skipped class, was drawn to the local party scene, and lacked self-esteem. Friends who took advantage of her kindness and loyalty hurt her time and again, and her fluctuating confidence was challenged in Army Cadets, when one minute she excelled and the next she was in "big trouble." At times, she was responsible, caring and funny but at home, we often caught her frustration, anger, pain and self-hatred. Her worrying and inability to sleep at night played havoc with routine. When she and her Dad called a truce and decided to go to Mexico, I was pleased. For them, it was a wonderful chance at some much needed healing in their erratic father-daughter relationship. They were both very intense people but perhaps in a holiday setting they could relax.

There was much to be thankful for. The sisters' relationship had improved from "You're a spoiled little brat," and "My big sister's so mean," to "My little sister's so cute," and "My big sister's cool." With almost eight years between them, there were bound to be some bumps in the road but this sudden change of attitude made for some welcome peace. Rachel's nurturing and creativity, and Becky's funny dry wit were finally shining through. We were making progress.

"Hey, Mom, I need some new reeds for my clarinet." Rachel played in the school and military band, more out of duty than a burning desire to play, but it was another disciplined creative outlet for her.

"I'm dreading marching this year on Canada Day. Maybe I'll quit by then. I'm fed up with the drama, and kids not showing up. Our band is shrinking." The four-kilometre walk dressed in full uniform during a hot July First morning quickly lost its glamour in the melting heat.

"Okay, let's just get a few reeds for now." She had already given up the school band, and I suspected the military band might fold. Rachel had started working part-time at Tim Horton's, and there were many demands on her time.

~~~~~~

One day at the pool, a lifeguard and I started talking about the value of nutrition in general health and energy.

"Because of MS, I really struggle with more tiredness than most people, although it's a common problem for all ages. My teenage daughter is often tired, people I work with are exhausted, and it seems everywhere I go people are tired. I'm fighting this with exercise, rest and mindful nutrition." The lifeguard nodded in understanding.

"You know, Kathy, I've started my family on something to help some of those issues, which we face too. Have you ever heard of *nutraceuticals?*"

"No, I haven't."

"They're products used to boost the immune system and promote health. Maybe it could help you."

"Is it a pill, like vitamins?" I knew the health food store in town had many such products.

"No, it's actually a powder that you can mix into juice, sprinkle on cereal and that sort of thing. I'm actually getting into selling it, and if you're interested, you could come to an information night I'm organizing."

"I'll think about it and let you know." I was a bit sceptical, but over the next few weeks investigated further by asking friends and reading the brochure Lisa had given me.

I agreed with the premise that poor nutrition, or inadequate nutrition, was a culprit behind many health problems including disease, so maybe this could help me. I also liked the idea of a natural rather than a chemical product to promote healing, even though I had opted for conventional drug treatment by using an interferon. Why couldn't the two work together?

I attended the promotion night that my friend arranged, and brought home samples to try. My biggest concern was the high cost, but knew I could tap into savings if I was convinced this was right for me. The testimonies were encouraging and I was able to read those written by people who had MS, with stories that ranged from miraculous healing to small noted improvements. I knew a couple of people at work taking the product who hadn't noticed huge differences in their health, but had found small, significant changes and more energy. Some friends were cynical and disbelieving, and many more had never heard of such a thing. I watched a video, read about the science behind it and all the literature that was available. There was no conflict with my current medication so I decided to try it.

It was difficult to tell if it was helping since my energy and tiredness were never predictable, but persisting was okay with me. It took a long time for the disease to register in my body, and perhaps the same would be true for "repairs."

At least I had adjusted easily enough to the medication. A few heart-stopping moments had occurred when insurers, doctors, and pharmacies had not coordinated the necessary paperwork, and I wondered how I would pay for it. Fortunately, it never came to that. Physically I still felt strong, unless I had to walk long distances or tried to pack too much activity into a day.

I had chosen the lowest dose of interferon, which statistically slowed the progression of MS by thirty percent. The neurologist recommended a higher dose but I wanted to start slowly. Doubling the dose only added a few percentage points.

Side effects were minimal. I noticed a huge thirst during the night and had a harder time waking up. The dark, freezing cold mornings did not help, but somehow we made it to school on time. Many days were so full that I could not always remember if I had injected myself the night before. I kept a journal to keep track of dates, the rotation of injection sites, when to order more medication and any other important details. A front and back drawing of the human body was a handy reference to the injection sites and helped me to avoid putting a needle in the same spot. I told myself I was lucky to have opportunity and provision for the interferon, but I did not feel lucky. A little voice reminded me to trust the bigger picture – I had hope and a future in that plan.

ELEVEN

"Change your thoughts and you
change your world."
~ Norman Vincent Peale ~

Our trip to the Dominican Republic was filled with adventure. We experienced plenty of relaxation, laughter, and fun but also had a few stresses like painful sunburns and post 9/11 airport treatment. In order to get the exact travel dates we needed, we ended up with an all-day flight schedule that involved changing planes several times, long jaunts across huge airports, and patience (not always my strong point).

Bernadette and a Dominican friend met us at the small airport in Puerto Plata, at the end of a very long day of travelling. Exhaustion, gratitude and exhilaration poured through my veins as I hugged my good friend.

"I'm so glad you're here! And you too, Becky, the boys can't wait to see you."

"Where are the boys?" Becky asked. She had just woken from another nap on the plane and had a new burst of energy. Bernadette laughed.

"They're with their Dad at the place where we're staying, probably sleeping."

"What time is it here?" I had lost all sense of time.

"About 11.30 pm"

"Oh my gosh, we got up at 5 am to catch the first plane." There was no point in figuring out the time change differences – we would adjust. I looked at the palm trees and exotic vegetation as we walked to the van, forgetting about my tiredness. I drew in a deep breath.

"It even smells exotic, and it's so warm! I can't wait for the morning to see it all."

"Where are we going?" Becky asked, as the van started moving.

"A place called Cabarete. It's a forty-five minute drive. Maybe when we get there you can go for a swim in the pool after all the sitting you've done today."

"Yaaaay, can I go swimming, Mom?"

"Of course, I might join you." A swim would be a perfect way to unwind.

"I hope you'll like the place, Kathy. It's very small, only eight suites, and not fancy at all. But it's clean, quiet and about four blocks from the ocean, away from the busy main road. We love it." It sounded just right for us.

The pool glistened in the center of the tiled courtyard in the dusky light of a huge full moon, surrounded by palm trees. Some suites were around the pool area and lounge chairs sat invitingly outside each door. I sighed. It was perfect.

"Mom, Mom, where's my bathing suit?" Becky could not wait to get in the pool, so I only glanced around at the small living room with kitchenette, separate bedroom and bathroom as I wiggled into my swimsuit. More tiles on the floors. I liked the simplicity.

"In your black bag, just dig deep."

The air outside was rich with moisture and I sat down on the pool steps as Becky plunged into the tranquil water. Bernadette sat beside the pool and lit a cigarette, smiling.

"Come in, Mom. It's warm." I sat on the edge of the

kidney-shaped pool for a minute longer, until a small splash of water hit my shoulder and trickled down my bathing suit.

"Okay, okay, here I come." I slowly descended the four stairs that led into the water. Becky took my hand and led me into the deep end, which was barely over my head at the furthest point. She paddled confidently to the edge and waited for me to return. We splashed and played together for a few minutes, and then I hauled myself out of the water and reached for a towel. I joined Bernadette and we talked while Becky splashed about.

"There's no rush to get moving in the morning, but when you're ready, we'll walk to the beach. Lyn and Rob will probably come too." Another couple, good friends from Calgary, had joined the holiday group.

Becky finally had her fill of water and we followed her into our suite as she dripped across the tiles. Bernadette looked around.

"I hope everything's okay. The only thing that doesn't work in this suite is the fridge, so you can use ours. We can buy some food tomorrow, or the owners serve breakfast if you're starving. It's really good, but we're trying to eat only one meal a day at a restaurant to keep expenses down, and we usually wait until dinner." Bernadette wandered into the bedroom in flip-flops and watched a centipede crawl along the wall. She whacked it with her sandal and deposited the unwanted creature outside in the trees. "Those are the only creepy crawlers around here that bother me. I stepped on one in the dark and it bit me, so make sure you wear something on your feet at night." Bernadette grimaced. This was not great news, but travelling in Mexico and Belize several times in the past had made me aware that bugs are part of the tropical experience.

"Thanks for the warning," I replied, making a face.

"You're welcome! I'll see you in the morning. Good-night, Becky." I gave my friend a big hug and we closed the door. Soon, everything was quiet and I drifted off to sleep listening to the rhythmic buzz of night creatures, broken occasionally by a loud, raucous cry, perhaps of a tropical bird. I was startled awake at first light by a sound familiar to me, and the "er-er-er-er-errrrr" of a rooster reminded me I was in a land where animals, people and nature blended by circumstance and climate, but not always in harmony. I listened to Becky's short, light breath beside me, and eventually fell back asleep, dreamless and still.

I woke up slowly, drifting in and out of consciousness, until an unfamiliar shriek brought me to my feet. Through our window, I could see trees with huge curling leaves, dangling vines, shrubs and thick vegetation. From the other window, all I saw was a wall of woven grass with a patch of blue in one corner. Becky was still sleeping so I padded to the bathroom before opening the door to the courtyard.

My eyes feasted on the dreamlike setting. The translucent water in the pool shimmered in the morning sunlight, shaded in places by palm and banana leaves. To the right, a thatched roof covered a small, open area with tables and chairs. I recognized the grass walls as the ones that faced our bedroom window. There was a quaint, single-storey house, a garage, and a gravel driveway. A low makeshift fence, finished with barbed wire, and a gate to the road partitioned off the property, including our suites and pool. A lone horse stood in the adjacent land, amidst more lush vegetation.

Tile, patio and grass were interspersed with exotic plants, and several "apartments" sat across from us, where our hosts slept. Bernadette sat quietly reading in a chair with a mug in hand, and I waved when I saw the boys coming out of their suite. We met in the middle of the courtyard and I gave them each a hug.

"Is Becky still sleeping?" Ben asked.

"She is. You can go and see for yourself. I'm going to visit with your mom." Bernadette offered me a welcome cup of coffee and we sat outside together, watching Becky follow the boys out of our suite, rubbing her eyes.

"Morning, sleepy head."

"Hi, Mom." The kids sat together on a patch of grass near the fence and started talking. A wicker chair with cushions hung suspended from a tree, which they took turns sitting in. I turned to Bernadette.

"Where's Andy?"

"He went to get some bread. Did you sleep well?"

"I had a great sleep. What a beautiful little spot! No wonder you wanted to come back." They had discovered the area over Christmas when school was out.

After a leisurely morning, introductions, and a special house breakfast, we headed off to the beach. Out of the protection of shady streets, my pace slowed, and we stopped at the busy corner market for some snacks and cold drinks. They would not stay cold for long.

Cars, trucks, taxis and motorcycles zipped by as we crossed the main road. We strolled towards the sand past colourful houses and a sight that stopped us in our tracks. Parked on the side of the road was a scooter, with a large partially gutted fish strapped to the back of the seat, dripping entrails and blood everywhere. One eye bulged out as silvery skin caught the suns rays. The long, smooth body lay perpendicular to the bike, head and tail drooped towards the ground, and unconcerned locals sauntered by with barely a glance, as we stood and fumbled for our cameras while the kids gawked.

At the beach, my legs were unsteady on the shifting sand and Bernadette proffered her arm, which I gratefully took. It made me think of the snow I had stumbled through in our backyard before we came. This was similar. What was happening to my balance? Once we were set up under an umbrella with a lounge chair, the kids ran to the water's edge, I relaxed somewhat and soon forgot about my wobbly legs.

Andy pointed to the far end of the fine, sandy beach.

"Look at the Para sailors in the sky!" A steady ocean breeze kept the bright sails aloft, and wind-surfers popped up and down in the strong waves. Restaurants, hotels, and palm trees sprawled over two kilometres of shoreline, and the kids ran about happily in the sun and water. Becky and I were badly sunburned so I vowed to be more vigilant about sun protection. It seemed I would never learn about the power of the sun.

In the early evening, tantalizing smells of local seafood drifted our way. In the glorious setting sun, we wandered down the beach and feasted on the biggest prawns I had ever seen. The butter and garlic enhanced their delicate flavour and we sopped up the juices with chunks of fresh bread. It was dark when we set out for home, bellies full and the children's eyes blinking to stay awake. We followed a little corridor up through some shops to the main road, and Bernadette suggested we catch a ride.

"Watch this." She stepped off the sidewalk, lifted her arm and wiggled a finger. Suddenly, a motorcycle driver wearing a vest pulled over and she spoke to him in Spanish.

"It's cheap. Let's take bikes home. We need two more," she said to Andy as they motioned more drivers to stop. I sandwiched Becky between the driver and me and we followed the others to our hotel. The kids were tired and it really helped conserve my energy, so we often returned from the beach via motorcycle. It was fun, too.

The days blended into one another in similar fashion. Becky and I explored the local shops, bought trinkets and soaked up the casual holiday atmosphere. The street was filled with interesting smells, blaring horns, laughter, yelling, locals dressed in bright, colourful clothing with contrasting dark skin that glowed in the hot sun. We wandered into a shop and I picked up a picture frame decorated with tiny seashells. I used my broken Spanish.

"Hola. Quanto para este?"

"Cincuenta pesos for you, miss." I wanted to practise speaking Spanish but found most of the shopkeepers had a good knowledge of English. It was usually possible to negotiate a price, and I enjoyed "bartering" with numbers, back and forth, until I was satisfied. I saw similar items in several stores but prices varied considerably, just like at home.

One day we took a cab to a nearby beach where snorkelling was supposed to be good. It was much smaller, packed with people, shops and open-air restaurants. The bay was protected from the powerful ocean and water was calm. The water danced with colours of aqua, lime green and blue-gray.

I struggled to get the snorkelling gear on. The mask was a poor fit and I knew a good seal was important. I tightened the straps and sat at the edge of the water to put on the flippers. Bernadette and Lyn were already in the water and I hurried to catch up, stumbling several times over my huge, webbed feet. When the water was over a foot deep, I clenched down on the mouthpiece and plunged in, pushing forcefully off the uneven ocean bottom toward deeper water.

I saw a new world under the calm surface. Little mountains of bumpy, dimpled rock stood beckoning and, as I approached, several red- and orange-striped fish swam by, disappearing into the murky depths of coral. There were sea sponges, anemones and schools of colourful fish. It appeared rather sparse in sea-life compared to my past snorkelling experiences in Mexico and Belize, but the longer I looked, the more I discovered subtly blended in and cleverly disguised as part of the undersea landscape. I watched a crab scurry away and a tiny octopus curling its long arms. Every so often, I checked for the shoreline and swam in to a depth where I could stand and empty out water that kept leaking into the mask. I soon passed my gear onto Andy and went to join the kids. The sand was hot under my feet.

The travelling merchants fascinated me. As well as jewellery and trinkets, peddlers brought fresh fruit, baked goods and cold drinks. In Cabarete, a large Dominican woman with dark, dark skin walked the beach each day carrying a large basket on her head, and one day I beckoned her over to see what she was selling.

It was local fruit, and I pointed to a large, ripe cantaloupe. We agreed on a price, I gave her the coin, and instead of handing me the fruit, she took out a large knife and began to cut expertly, exposing ripe orange flesh. She scooped out the seeds and began to cut wedges as sticky juice poured off the fruit into the sand, somehow balancing the entire thing on her hand as she worked. She held out a piece for me and placed the remainder into a large, plastic bag as I bit into my first piece. It was unlike any I had ever tasted - delicately sweet, delicious and dripping.

"Gracias, gracias," I said, as she packed up her wares.

"De nada. Buenos dias." She walked to the water's

edge and rinsed off, lifted the heavy basket onto her head and continued on, hips swaying, with sandaled feet, humming to herself.

Bernadette told me I could get a cantaloupe in the market for a third of the price. I didn't care. The experience is etched in my mind. I felt like a queen being served a royal delicacy in a beautiful land, honoured and humbled at the same time. Maybe I was helping to feed her family.

The week together passed all too quickly. Bernadette and family caught the bus back to Santo Domingo where she worked while her friends, Becky, and I had two more days of holiday before flying home. The following day, we decided to explore further along the island so we rented a car to get to our destination, Mount Isabel de Torres. The rules of the road were non-existent, but once past busy towns, we sped along and took a detour through a giant, sweet smelling cornfield. It was an amazing trip.

A gondola took us up the mountain for a spectacular view of the shoreline. We waited eons for a ride. A loud, enthusiastic band with guitars and banjos sang Spanish songs so it was impossible to talk in the large, clammy, space. Eventually we walked on a magical mountaintop in the clouds. A statue resembling the famous "Christ the Redeemer" statue in Rio de Janeiro, Brazil, stood with outstretched arms. Restored gardens with walkways abounded. Trails tempted visitors into the lush, tropical rainforest that stretched southward. I could almost taste the humidity in the moist, cool air and took picture after picture. We lingered near the gondola.

Overheating would have been a problem without the cooling ocean breeze, water, shade, hotel pool, fans and evening rest from the sun, triggering my debilitating MS symptom of fatigue. Four blocks to the ocean in the hot, tropical sun was my limit, although rest and shade seem to revive me. The distances I could walk were shrinking.

From the tarmac in Puerto Plata that afternoon, to the Edmonton airport the following day, the journey home had some surprises. We were delayed from the start, the flight across the Atlantic Ocean was turbulent and filled with bumps and heart stopping drops in elevation that frightened me. Passengers cried out in fear and a woman a few seats away from us began praying a long litany of Spanish that caused more people to panic. Then we missed our connecting flight in New York. After a thorough interrogation in Customs, we were forced to stay, stuck overnight in a very expensive hotel, at our cost. The airline refused to take responsibility for the initial delay – it was a baggage transportation problem in the previous country. Confusion prevailed and I cried at the check- in counter until I saw Becky's tired face.

"Mom, don't cry. We'll catch a plane tomorrow like the lady said." My seven-year-old was consoling a forty-two-year-old. I began a giddy laugh.

"Okay, you're right. I don't know why I'm crying. I guess I was looking forward to being home."

"I didn't really want to ride on another plane today, anyway. Where are we going now?" Becky sighed.

"First we collect our luggage, then we take a shuttle bus to our hotel. Hey, Becky, we're in New York, a really famous city. Maybe we'll see the Statue of Liberty or Ground Zero." I took her hand and we marched off.

We did not see a lot. It was dark, rainy, and we froze in our shorts. At least the hotel was close, and the rest of the flights went as scheduled. We got home to sunny skies and melting snow. I rolled down the window as we drove through the city and the smell of dog poop offended my nose repeatedly. Spring was on the way.

I had two more days off and felt rested, refreshed and ready to go back to work. Within a week, I was exhausted and lived week-end to week-end, when I could sleep more and set my own pace. I tried reducing commitments outside the home, going to bed earlier during the week, eating simple meals more often (we had got into the bad habit of drive-through restaurants), and being less picky about cleaning the house, vehicle and yard. Nothing I did made the intense tiredness disappear.

My neurologist convinced me to try a higher dose of interferon, which involved more forms, phone calls, faxes and letters. It was a mistake. After five months of torturous sleep filled with chills, shaking, sweating, nausea and dehydration, I switched back to the lower dose. The side effects were making life intolerable.

I discussed the possibility of working fewer hours at the school with the psychologist, neurologist and a few trusted friends. Our extended healthcare plan had provision for situations like mine, which I carefully considered before applying. I would receive seventy percent of my wages to cover the lost hours and would be paid for the remainder I worked, which seemed like a small sacrifice to make for the rest time I so desperately needed. This development had surprised me even though all the signs had been there. I had carried on despite the falls. Was it denial, stupidity, and stubbornness or was I just crazy? I applied for "accommodation employment," prepared for another round of appointments, phone calls and letters, and held my breath. I would not know until autumn if I had been approved.

In May, a crinkled brown package arrived in the mail, and I excitedly ripped at the paper, wondering what my aunt had sent from Vancouver. My fingers brushed soft cotton. I held up a white T-shirt with the words "THE SUPERCITIES 2003 WALK FOR MS" on the front, with about eighty sponsors listed on the back. My elderly aunt had walked five kilometres in North Vancouver with her daughter, Barb, fund raising for MS research. I wore the T-shirt with great pride.

For two summer months, I rested but unlike the past, when my energy would slowly recharge like a low battery, I only regained a portion of the total. I paced myself and paid for any overexertion by needing to sleep or sit for longer periods. This resulted not from deliberate exercise, but everyday activity like shopping, errands, cooking, cleaning and even showering. At least camping with my cousins was relaxing without the responsibility of children and I lazed about enjoying the water, eating huge ice cream cones and cooking on an open fire.

Travelling with my medication was a bit awkward, as it needed to be refrigerated. I used a special travel kit with icepacks, or threw it in the cooler if I was using one. Finding a private place to inject was sometimes a problem but I refused to let it stop me from trying new things. The bathroom at the campground had running water, showers and flush toilets, so this made the procedure manageable.

Kelly-Leigh came to Hinton for a few days at the end of August when the girls were home from their summer activities. The weather was gorgeous. Kelly-Leigh wanted to hike, camp and spend a few days in Jasper National Park. We discussed a few ideas.

"Is Mount Edith Cavell very close to Jasper? She was a heroine, you know. Listen to this." Kelly-Leigh held the book high and read:

"Described as the most impressive peak in Alberta,

203

Mt. Edith Cavell is named for a British nurse who was executed for treason after helping prisoners-of-war escape from Germany during World War 1. The peak is more than 11,000 feet tall and remains snow covered year round."

I nodded. "I think I've been up the access road years ago. It's not far from Jasper."

"Is there hiking on the mountain?" We both loved mountains and nature. Kelly-Leigh's strong feminist side adored female pioneers. They were women who had showed that through strength, determination and hard work, our country could be built step by step.

"There's a perfect shorter hike that Becky and I could do if you and maybe Rachel just want to hang out and relax in the parking area. My hiking guide says to allow one hour each way for Cavell Meadows, which takes us through alpine to Angel Glacier and Cavell Meadows Summit. It's supposed to be quite beautiful."

I knew I could not attempt the hike, but it did not matter, because parking area vistas were spectacular and a short jaunt up a wide, gravelled trail offered wonderful opportunities for photography with clear, sunny skies. Rachel sat alone in the car reading, feet draped casually out of the back window.

After a delicious campfire dinner of grilled steak, rice and vegetables, my friend settled down comfortably and opened a book. She started to read familiar words.

"There are strange things done in the midnight sun
By the men who moil for gold
The Artic Trails have their secret tales
That would make your blood run cold;"

Robert Service joined the party, and Kelly-Leigh's voice changed in pitch and tone as she made the lines come to life. She tapped the book and laughed deeply.

"You should have seen your Grandpa, Becky, reciting this poem. It was amazing. Let's do it again!"

She started before any of us could protest. Kelly-Leigh paused suddenly and pointed to us. Becky caught on right away. "Sam McGee," she shouted and soon we were all chiming his name at the right time and smiling at each other.

Becky loved it and wanted more. Rachel was less enthusiastic, but it had at least brought her out of her shell of silence. The next day we went on a beginner white water rafting trip on the Athabasca River. We were jostled and splashed just enough to make it memorable.

I was sad to see summer end. The weather continued warm and pleasant, and after hours spent organizing, sorting, and shopping, I rested on a reclining lawn chair in the shade, sipping tea and reading. The pictures from the Jasper trip sat beside me on the table. As I dozed fitfully my mind slipped back in time.

~~~~~~

At Manning Park, east of Hope, we piled out of the bus into the park building for snacks and bathroom breaks. It was almost dark, but I barely noticed. Delays seemed to be part of life, and besides, I was going on my first overnight hike with friends in a provincial park.

The bus took forever to climb the mountain, slowing down at each sharp turn. We chatted excitedly as the teacher gave instructions for the two-kilometre walk to the first camp.

"The trail is well marked and only steep in a couple of spots. I'll lead and Miss Brown will bring up the rear, so you don't have to worry about being left behind. We'll set up our tents when we get there and leave the rest until morning." Everyone clapped.

I adjusted my heavy metal-framed backpack and set out on

the trail. The partial moon offered a bit of light, but I soon lost track of the student in front of me. I tripped over something hard, fell to my side, quickly stood up and went on, brushing myself off as I walked. The straps were biting into my shoulders. I fell again and this time the pack cushioned my fall. I frowned. By the third fall, I was frustrated. The palms of my hands stung and I swore under my breath.

"You all right, Kathy?" Miss Brown asked me as she came down the trail.

"Yeah, I'm okay. I keep falling, though, which is kind of strange."

"It's late, dark and an unfamiliar trail. You're probably just tired." That had to be it, because the next day I did not fall once and we hiked for ten kilometres.

~~~~~~

I awoke with a start. I had not thought about that hike and all those falls for years. Could that have been MS? No one else fell as much as I did. I was 16 years old, in grade eleven.

Approval to work part-time came in early September. It was a blessed relief and quietened some of my anxiety. In my excitement, I filled the first couple of months with activities I liked - baking, reading, and working on my writing course. Sometimes, though, I walked through the door ready to fall over. One day I finally gave in and lay down on the couch - three hours later I awoke groggy and stiff. How could I have slept so long? I continued this pattern and found it was a challenge to keep the time to an hour (otherwise I could not get to sleep at night when I needed to) because I often ignored my alarm and continued sleeping while the rest of the world was busy working, doing and accomplishing things. I banished the guilt because my body demanded it. Sleep was pure bliss and when I closed my eyes, it came almost instantly. Extra stiffness seemed to accumulate during this rest, mostly in my legs and back, but I could not stop the changes.

Once the cold winter began, my feet were never warm. Shovelling the gravel driveway became a big chore and my retired neighbour often took the time to plough what snow he could out of the way. I learned to do only the essentials and leave the rest alone.

I hated admitting it, but passing Melissa on to another more physically capable teacher assistant was a good decision for me. It was hard to let her go because we had spent three years together but the time had come for me to be realistic. I was assigned to a grade four classroom to give support in whatever way was needed. I sat whenever possible, used the elevator to the second floor, and found my stress level much reduced. The migraines subsided. I had been on an interferon for almost a year with no adverse effects except continuing red spots around the injection sites.

~~~~~~

One Sunday morning at church as people mingled and visited in the large foyer, sipped coffee and ate goodies I turned towards the kitchen and caught my left foot on the carpet, lunged forward and tried frantically to regain my balance. My arms flew out and I grabbed the first thing in sight - a ten-year old boy. Fortunately, I did not pull him down with me. I stood up and lurched out the back door, appalled at myself. My mouth was dry.

I sat in my cold vehicle and I thought about what I should do - apologize. I forced myself to return, made amends quickly, and retreated. My confidence was draining as the falls were beginning to threaten others as well as myself. What would happen if I pulled a child down with me at school? I recalled the surprise of pulling a clothing rack over while shopping one day and falling flat on my face in the hallway at school. There had been no witnesses to these random events and at the time, I had been grateful, but maybe I needed to be "shaken" out of my fear.

Rachel's relationship with her Dad continued to be distant and rocky. She did not seem comfortable around adults. Becky, on the other hand, was happy to go to Robb about once a month to spend a weekend. Dave called on Wednesday night to confirm a visit.

"Okay, any time after school on Friday works fine." I looked forward to the weekends when I had a break from being full-time mom.

"Kathy, did you know Steven Desrosiers is sick again? He's been in the hospital in Edmonton for quite a while. Dawn and Bruno are getting really worn out from trips to the city."

"I'm sorry to hear that. I know the past few years have been really hard."

"Yes. Well, I'll see Becky on Friday, then. Bye." Dawn's kids were her priority, but the weakest one required more and more of her time and energy. Steven had been in and out of hospital for most of his short life, and they had almost lost him a couple of times. She never gave up and remained by Steven's side.

Dave phoned again on Valentine's Day.

"Steven passed away yesterday. I thought you'd like to know." I had already heard the sad news but appreciated Dave's call. He was good friends with Steven's parents. My girlfriend had called with the news hours before, and I was stunned. Death was like that. You thought you were prepared, but it was too final, overwhelming and heart breaking.

The funeral was held in Robb on February 19th. Dave mentioned how distraught Dawn was about who might speak about their oldest son, and I recalled the year I was Steven's teacher assistant, voice, advocate and support. I had spent time getting to know Steven on a human, intimate level, and respected his courage to get through a day. I stepped out of my comfort zone and offered to give a eulogy of Steven's life. His parents were very grateful and the words poured onto paper straight from my heart. Speaking it was much harder, but I wanted to help Steven's family in their grief, so I pushed my nervousness aside. It was not too bad. Dawn's tired, drawn face shone as I read the words and I knew I had helped in some small way.

Spring break came, and we followed through with our plans to fly to Vancouver and spend a week visiting family and friends. It had been too long since all three of us had spent any time in the place I grew up. I ignored Rachel's less than enthusiastic response.

We had to make the three-hour drive east on Saturday morning to catch our plane. Rachel did not pack a bag but went out with her friends on Friday night. I had trouble getting to sleep worrying about her disinterest. On Saturday morning, I heard her come in and rolled over to look at the clock. It was 7 am. I heard Rachel crashing around in her bedroom and realized she was packing.

I dozed off and awoke to find Rachel passed out on the couch in the living room. I warned her we were leaving in an hour and she groaned. At least it was not snowing or minus thirty, I thought as Becky and I had breakfast and took care of last-minute details.

"Rachel, we're leaving in a few minutes. Are you ready?"

"Whaaaat? I don't want to go." She mumbled from under the blanket.

"Well, you don't have a choice. I've already booked

you a plane ticket, and your relatives haven't seen you for four years." I told myself she would snap out of it. "You can sleep in the truck."

"I'm not going." I took a deep breath, and continued to get ready. In my mind, she did not have a choice. At nine o'clock, I started the engine and roused her.

"Time to go, Rachel. I put your bag in the truck."

"Maaahom, I told you, I don't want to go. It's spring break and all my friends get to sleep in and party while I'm gone. It's not fair." She got up and stomped outside, bringing her suitcase into the house.

"You're going. I've already paid for the flight." I marched her bag back out to the car and waited a few minutes, but she did not move. My stomach was churning.

"Rachel, we're going to miss the plane. You can't stay here by yourself, anyway." The clock was moving fast and the extra time I had allowed for "unexpected delays" was being gobbled up.

Finally, she went out to the truck and threw herself in the backseat. Becky was sitting quietly in the front with her seatbelt on.

"I don't want to go and be dragged all over Vancouver to see relatives I don't even know any more. I'll make your trip miserable."

"I bet you will." I could not believe this was happening. We were going to miss the plane if I did not make a decision.

"I'll be fine. A friend could stay with me. You had better hurry up, or you'll miss your plane." She grabbed her bag and went inside the house. I followed her.

"Did you plan this last minute strategy? You've done this before." I was shaking with anger and frustration. If I waited any longer none of us would go, never mind Rachel. If I forced Rachel to come, I had no doubt she would make the week miserable. I backed out of the driveway. Becky started to cry.

"I'm sorry, Becky. It's better this way. We'll have a much better time without Rachel to complain and be grouchy. Don't cry."

The trip was filled with disappointment. I had made arrangements to stay with my brother Paul the first night and looked forward to spending a few hours with him in person but Paul, in his usual nervous style, ran out on us an hour after we arrived.

"I'm sorry, Kath. I have to leave a day earlier than I thought on this business trip. You know how it is. But I want to you to make yourselves at home and stay as long as you like." He left.

My temples throbbed. We had come to spend time with family and so far, two members had bailed out. I called Mike. He and his wife convinced me to drive the rental car (in the rainy dark night across the city) to their home, an hour away. Eddie said if we did not come to them, she would come and get us. I forced myself to move. It was the best thing we could have done. Becky had her cousins to play with and I had company.

It was a work and school week for them, and their busy schedule did not allow much downtime. I had not thought about that very carefully, and figured we would be off doing things in the city so it would not matter, but it was not relaxing. It rained everyday, traffic was horrendous and I was concerned about Rachel. On the trip home, someone took my suitcase by mistake and on the drive home, it snowed and roads were slippery.

I dragged our bags inside and the door slammed behind me. The cat ran away.

"Hi, Rachel, we're home!" Rachel came out of her room a minute later.

211

"Hi, Mom, how was your trip?" She was surprisingly pleasant.

"It was okay. How did your week go?" She rummaged around in the fridge.

"My week was good. We don't have much food, though." I glanced in the near empty fridge. Mail was piled neatly on the table, and the cat dishes were full. The house looked reasonably clean at a glance, and I could smell the pine scent of cleanser. The phone rang.

"Hi, I was wondering if you were missing a suitcase. I accidentally pulled the wrong one off the carousel and didn't notice until I got home. I'm terribly sorry. It'll be on the next Greyhound bus." The black suitcase arrived intact, but I discovered Becky's birth certificate had gone missing.

Within twenty-four hours, I realized things were not quite as they seemed around our house.

"Rachel, where's the sugar dish? The floor is really sticky in spots. And what happened to this chair?" She avoided my eyes.

"Mom, the dish got broken, and so did the chair. I'm sorry. I tried to glue it. I threw the dish away."

"How did the chair get broken?" The dish I could understand, but the chair?

"Umm, I had a few people over last Saturday night, and that's when it broke." She disappeared into her room.

Over the next few days, I made more discoveries. My neighbours told me the police had been to the house and a teacher mentioned her son had been to a party on our street the weekend before. I found a few more broken items and a small dent in the drywall in the kitchen. The remote control for the television was missing and there were new stains on the carpet. The fire pit out back was heaped with charred wood and my aluminum lawn chair I used for camping was gone.

Rachel and I had a big talk. Apparently, it started out as a small party, but soon kids Rachel did not know were walking in the door and things got a "little crazy." She was sorry.

She paid for the missing and broken items. She was not allowed to stay at our house if I was out of town and she did more repairs and cleaning. Communication between us was strained, and I could hardly wait until she went to cadet camp for six weeks in the summer. I wanted to kick her out. I felt like a failure as a parent.

Talking to other parents, our youth pastor, friends at work, Rachel's teachers, and counsellors, offered a broader perspective. It was a scary time for me and for Rachel. I wondered if she would graduate. She did not seem to care about anything the adult world considered important.

~~~~~~

Our school held a spring dance for its students on a Friday evening late in May. The week had been full, and I could not wait to put my feet up and do nothing. Becky frowned.

"Aaaawh, Mom, I really, really want to go to this dance. You just have to drive to the school parking lot and walk to the gym. You can sit the whole time."

"Uh-huh. I have this problem, Becky. My legs have no strength left in them. I can barely walk." Becky started to cry, which did not happen very often.

"I promised my friends I'd be there, and I need to have a parent with me. Please, Mom, I'll hold your arm," Becky pleaded. I thought of the black cane sitting uselessly in the closet.

"I could try using my cane."

"Yes, if that would work, then I could go!"

"You wouldn't care if I walked in the school with it?"

I had gone to physiotherapy five months before for instruction on using the cane correctly, but hid it away soon after, sceptical and ashamed of my "weakness." I knew it was a self-defeating, wrong way for me to think but I just could not shake the feeling. I was not ready for the label.

Scripture said, "In your weakness, I am strong" and "With faith, nothing shall be impossible for you." I needed faith, my cane, and Becky's need, to move me forward figuratively, literally and practically. It was simple.

Why did I hate the cane so much? It was going to help me, not hurt me. I took a deep breath. If it took desperation, I guess that is what I needed. The support of the cane made a huge difference and I was able to walk across the street and into the school.

I was grateful for the dark room. The kids who saw me every day at school gave me some puzzled looks, open stares and asked questions. It was hard to explain, especially in that atmosphere, so I said I had a disease that made my legs weak. The kids accepted the explanation but I knew there would be further queries in the halls from many who had seen me walk just fine before. I was crossing a line I did not want to cross.

The summer was a welcome relief in my new situation of "sometimes disabled." I started using my cane on a regular basis whether I needed it or not, because eventually I really did need it as the day progressed and I got tired of the questions "Where's your cane?" and "Why do you need that?" It was a huge adjustment for a person who was used to having a lot of energy and being capable and physically strong. A good way to cope was to crack a joke or two. I offered my cane to a few teachers at work during assembly for "crowd control" and "shepherding." Eventually I let the kids bring it to me and nothing was funnier than watching a ten-year-old pretend limp down the hall, leaning on the cane. If I did not laugh, I would cry.

It was time to find a hobby that was restful so when I received a brochure in the mail, "Writing for Children," I decided it was a good fit for me and signed up for the correspondence course. It was exciting to start doing something I had wanted to do for years. I told myself I needed to do this and had to stop making excuses or it would never happen. It was a dream to fulfill.

I was struggling with feelings I did not quite understand. I cried a lot, felt over-whelmed, and had trouble staying positive. When I thought about it, I realized that tears had come far too often in the past year. After some deliberation, I decided to try an anti-depressant. The neurologist said it might help the fatigue as well.

~~~~~~

Becky and I travelled to Ontario to visit Kelly-Leigh. The night before we left, I fell, stepping through the back door. Tripping over the ledge, I flew across the eight-foot room into the wall and fell hard on my left knee, getting the worst "rug-burn" ever, deep and painful. I still have a scar. It was amazing I was not more injured, but I picked myself up and carried on. This was an important trip for us because I was going to see people I had not seen for years, people who meant a lot to me and who were going out of their way to make our trip the best.

We spent time in Waterloo and visited the shores of Lake Huron where we swam and soaked in the sun. We had a bonfire on the beach and recited more Robert Service poetry. Ontario is a beautiful province in the summer, with rich green hills, a huge variety of trees and flowers, lakes, and small communities around every corner. We were lucky enough to spend time in Collingwood, Lindsay and Balsam Lake. I met Pierre, Kelly-Leigh's new man, her parents, my Uncle Bill, cousins and their families. Kelly-Leigh entrusted me with the keys to her BMW and Becky and I drove the infamous 401 Highway, happy to be alive. We got lost (a lot), were late by several hours (a few times), but eventually got where we wanted. It was all worth it.

Adjusting to the anti-depressant was tricky and it spoiled many a sleep for me until I figured out a "formula" that my body could handle. The very lowest dose did nothing and the next available level caused disturbing side effects. I could not get to sleep. When I finally did, I soon woke up and the cycle started all over again.

The worst part was that the drug dulled my extreme feelings. In fact, it deadened them. It really took away my enjoyment of life. I lived with it for a few months and then one day forgot to take a pill. The next day something sad happened and I felt tears come to my eyes. They were real tears, but not the racking-my-body, out-of-control kind of tears that made me feel so helpless. I realized that was the formula. I tried taking a pill every second day and the system worked beautifully. My depression remained in check, but I could still feel my emotions. I finally felt somewhat balanced.

In August, while camping in the Okanagan, my bowel and bladder played a few tricks on me. I kept my "accidents" a secret, ashamed to share my latest embarrassing episodes. There were some unusual stressors, such as extreme heat, construction noise, and shared bathrooms that were a few minutes walk from our campsite, locked from 11 pm until 7 am. There was an outhouse to use in the interim. I tried to anticipate my needs, but it did not always work. I joked to myself about getting some "Depends," adult incontinence wear, but fortunately things settled down and I only had to live with infrequent flare-ups. It was humbling. I remembered my Dad's major episode with colitis, and could now imagine the mental and emotional anguish that he suffered.

Work remained a challenge but I was determined to adapt. In the fall, I was assigned to another grade four classroom, where Becky was placed.

"Will it bother you if I work in your classroom, Becky?" I was not sure about mother and daughter together, but it proved to work well. My focus was on a boy who had behaviour problems and we spent a lot of time together.

"That's fine, Mom. I'm happy that Madi and Mickey are in my class. And I really like my teacher, Mr. Schroder." I was enjoying Ron's experienced teaching style. He was firm, caring and funny, and I looked to him for leadership in helping Nick. Ron had a reputation for handling these problem kids well without compromising his values or over-involving the rest of the class. Nick was bright and charming but his quick anger, sneaky ways, and lack of focus presented a challenge. I tapped into his creative, funny side to help him in language arts, and he responded very well to begin with as we read together in the large storage room at the back of the classroom.

A few months passed and Nick began to experience conflict with other kids. Some bullying behaviour at recess put him in the principal's office several times. Ron stepped up the consequences as Nick's behaviour escalated and he became almost hyperactive. We added another student to the language arts lesson in the back room to try to add some balance and help the other boy

217

with his skills. I was giving the boys a modified spelling test one Friday morning.

"Nick, sit down, please, and get ready for your words. Did you study?"

"No, I forgot. But I know them anyway." He left the room and I decided to go ahead and test the other student, who had different words than Nick. I stood up and began to recite the list slowly.

"Stopped. He stopped the car. Stopped." The door stood ajar, and I could hear Ron reading the spelling words Becky had studied briefly that week. Nick suddenly burst in, pushing the door hard.

"Started. She started to cr..." I sailed into boxes stacked against the wall, doing an odd little dance waving my arms wildly and stiffening my legs to stop the fall that, surprisingly, never came. I hit my elbow hard on the table and hurt my shoulder.

"Sorry, Ms. M., I didn't know you were there." Nick sat down and I stared at him. Ron heard the commotion.

"Everything okay in here? Nick, you can't just run out whenever you feel like it."

"But I had to go to the bathroom. Can I write my test now?" Nick looked at me as I sat gingerly on a chair. We carried on, but I stood well away from the door after that. A few trips to the chiropractor eased my sore back, and when the bruises disappeared, I treated myself to a massage. As my tense body relaxed and muscles were kneaded under skilled hands, my mind relaxed too.

~~~~~~

The birdie flew across the net, and I lunged forward to make contact before it dropped to the ground. My partner had the same strategy and we met in the middle of the court.

"Wham." The metal racquet came down hard on my wrist and pain shot up my arm as I fell to the floor. My arm was numb, with a dull throbbing where my partner's racquet had

hit and I reached out with useless fingers that refused to grip.

"Sorry, Kathy. Are you okay? I guess we both wanted that birdie to go back where it came from." He helped me up, and nausea overwhelmed me. I staggered to the bench and sat down.

"I'll sit this one out. Maybe Marlene could play."

My arm continued to tingle and throb, and I left, barely noticing the badminton players who stood ready.

TWELVE

"Two are better than one...if one falls
down, the other can help him up."
~ Ecclesiastes 4:9-10 ~

We had a new cat named "Bubbles" join our family. Missy was not very impressed, but they soon got used to each other and did not fight much. Bubbles was a good-natured cat who liked everyone, and I enjoyed her company when she curled up beside me on the couch. The only thing we did not like were the presents she brought home - dead mice, birds and even squirrels fell prey to her quick-moving body and sharp claws. I put a bell on her collar but it did not slow her down much.

Rachel was in grade twelve, her last year of high school. She quit Army Cadets.

"I can't believe I'm almost finished. There's a lot to do this year with fund-raisers and grad planning. We're selling a bunch of food items, and I'm auditioning for the fashion show. And grad photos are really early, in a couple of months, and I really, really want a grad ring." I was warned by my friends that graduation year was very expensive, but the more Rachel fund-raised, the less our tickets would cost for the formal dinner scheduled in May. It was being held at Jasper Park Lodge and had been an annual tradition for many years. To add to the excitement, Rachel had her learner's permit to drive, and was scheduled to take a driver's education class.

We decided to take a "road trip" to Edson one Saturday to visit a close friend of Rachel's who was a bit older and had two little girls. I handed Rachel the keys.

"You drive. It's a good opportunity to get some highway driving experience." Rachel turned east on the Yellowhead Highway and we left the mountains behind us. She was confident and at ease behind the wheel.

"I don't know what happened, Rachel, but you have a different attitude this year. You're positive, and you seem to care more about everything. Before, you lived day-to-day, weekend-to-weekend, sick of school. Now that it's finally going to end, I guess you see things from a new angle."

"I feel different. It's finally my turn to choose what I want for the future. I think I'd like to get out of this town, and maybe travel."

"You'll get a whole new perspective if you do. There's no rush, though." I was enjoying the "new" Rachel and could not believe what a big change had occurred. If she was growing up at seventeen, what would she be like at twenty-one?

Over spring break, both daughters and I travelled to Lake Louise to meet Kelly-Leigh for the girls annual ski holiday. It was warm and sunny, and I enjoyed strolling along the paths to the shops, stopping for tea at the bakery, reading, resting and relaxing by the pool. We were so blessed to have such a generous friend.

We had a couple days left when we arrived home to get organized for the final stretch of the school year. I was sitting on my bed with the pillows propped up, finishing a poem that I was writing about Ron, who had been nominated for a teaching award through APPEGA (Association of Professional Engineers, Geologists and

Geophysicists of Alberta), when Rachel knocked on the door.

"Come in." Rachel sat down on the bed and frowned.

"What's up, Rach?"

"Amy blew it. Her aunt kicked her out. She says she's going to move to Cochrane where her Mom lives. How will she graduate?"

"That's a tough one, Rachel. She's so close to the end." Rachel had shared with me Amy's frustration about not being able to please her aunt but I knew she was a party girl and not always responsible. In addition, she struggled in school.

"Hey, Mom, do you think she could stay with us? It's only three more months, and she has almost the same schedule as me. She works at A&W too, so she wouldn't be broke and around all the time." Rachel looked imploringly at me.

"I'll have to think about it. It's a big decision for me." Could I manage one more kid? Could I afford it? How could I *not* help a kid who was so close to graduating?

A few days later, I told Rachel Amy could move her stuff in. Becky liked Amy and said it was fine with her. So we all agreed.

"There's just one thing, Amy. You have to promise to go to class, get your work done, and graduate from high school. I know you can do it."

"Oh, I will. And thanks for letting me stay with you guys."

The graduation party was held in Jasper, in May, on a cold Saturday. I could see my breath when I walked outside, although the sun was trying to break through. The girls looked so grown up in their long gowns, fancy hair-do's and heels. I barely recognized the guys in suits. The graduation class was transformed from denim-clad kids in T-shirts to young adults waiting to take on the world. With the backdrop of majestic mountains and the frozen lake, the grads looked ready for adventure and excitement, shivering in the cold crisp air for a class picture. We took family pictures inside the warm, elegant Lodge and the students milled about in small groups, talking and laughing. Amy sat with us for dinner. When speeches and awards started, the girls disappeared to join their graduating class. (The diploma part of the graduation was held separately, later in the year, after final exams were completed and marks tallied.)

The after-grad party was an all-night affair, which was our cue to exit. As we drove home, Becky fell asleep. A snowstorm swirled around us. I gripped the steering wheel hard as visibility diminished and the lines on the road disappeared. We slept late the next morning.

~~~~~~

I dreaded June. There were so many windup activities. Our students had exams, field trips, special event days like track and field, birthday parties, year-end parties, and class. The adults were part of most of that and had retirement parties, farewell parties, report cards and teaching to contend with. Some of it was exciting, some was fun, some was obligation and tradition, but for me, it was exhausting. I could hardly wait for the end of June to arrive. Maybe they would have to carry me out to my car.

In the meantime, after a check-up, my local doctor informed me I had high cholesterol.

"Well, we could put you on medication or you could try lowering your LDL with diet."

"What's LDL?"

"It stands for low density lipoprotein, and is typically referred to as 'bad fat.' HDL is a high-density lipoprotein, also called 'good fat.'"

"I'll try to lower the bad fat with diet first." After a bit of research, I ordered a copy of "Dr. Swank's Low Fat Diet" and eliminated baked goods, red meat, butter and chocolate from my regime. How did people survive diets? Ten months later, we retested and to my chagrin, the bad cholesterol had gone up. I was told I had probably inherited the tendency and I opted for a drug solution, something called a statin, which eventually lowered my bad LDL and raised the good HDL. I learned that statins are the most commonly prescribed drug to manage high cholesterol.

I asked my doctor about the handicapped parking stalls I had begun to notice in many parking lots. I realized it would shorten the distance I needed to walk and would help alleviate some of the exhaustion I felt after running errands and shopping. She immediately filled out a form and, through the local Motor Vehicle Branch, I soon had a three-year pass. It turned my disability into ability and made a tremendous difference to my confidence. I wanted to remain mobile.

The last day of school was warm and cloudless. We met in the gymnasium for the final assembly of the school year. I sat on the edge of my seat waiting for Ron to receive the teaching award some of us knew he was going to receive. When he was called up, the engineer from the industry presenting the award (the local mill) read some of the comments written in praise of Ron's teaching excellence in science and math. The first eight lines of the poem I wrote to nominate Ron were read first and I smiled. Many rave reviews and portrayals spoke of a dedicated, committed teacher. Ron was completely surprised. His wife and daughter sat proudly in the audience. We clapped and clapped. It was one of my favourite years at the school - I had learned a lot from Ron. We both valued children, family, faith, a positive outlook and poetry.

At the end of June, I met with my neurologist and we discussed my health concerns. Fatigue was wearing me down.

"There are a few medications that could help. You could try Amantadine or Alertec. Let me know and I can prescribe one for you anytime."

"I think I'll wait since summer break is starting and I should be able to get lots of rest." All I wanted to do was sleep off the tiredness. I also wanted to scream in frustration. "It feels like the stiffness is getting worse, too. I understand marijuana is supposed to help some of these symptoms." I had heard about pot helping some people and that there was a pill form.

"Marijuana is used more for treatment of pain. Do you have a lot of pain?" I hesitated in my response.

"Well, I don't have sharp shooting pain of any kind. I just have that weird tingly feeling in my legs and numbness in my feet."

"There are medications specifically for stiffness (spasticity), like Baclofen or Neurontine, but exercise also helps."

"Hmmm... I'll try and ride my bike more. I tend not to swim as much during the summer."

"I was thinking more of a daily stretching program. The physiotherapist could give you specific exercises and help you get started." I followed this recommendation and found fifteen minutes a day worked well for me. Even though it did not correct the "foot drop" I had developed from nerve damage in the lower left leg, which caused me to drag my foot and trip, I felt better. I ignored the suggestion of a brace, remembering Steven's torturous use of two full leg braces to try to help him stand.

In the local paper, I answered an ad for bike

maintenance and repair. I told the young man what I needed.

"I have problems with strength in my left leg, and my foot keeps slipping off the pedal after I start riding."

"Sounds like you could use toe-clips. I might have a few. I'll bring them with me."

Soon I was fixed up with a metal and plastic housing on the left pedal. I set out on a warm sunny afternoon to try out the new hardware. I walked the bike across the gravel driveway to the street, slid onto the seat, shoved my left foot into the toe-clip, and attempted to pedal forward. "Crash." The bike went down hard on the concrete, carrying me with it. My lip stung, and I tasted blood. The helmet I was wearing protected my head, but shorts left my legs exposed. "Owww. What the heck." I struggled to raise the bike up enough so I could get my foot out of the toe-clip. My knee was bleeding, and I limped with the bike into the backyard. I pulled out some paper towel and dabbed at my knee, sitting on the concrete step looking at the bike I had leaned carefully on the kickstand. What was I doing wrong?

I tried a few different ways of starting out and soon realized I needed some momentum with a slight decline, or a push. More importantly, the right foot needed to be in the raised position and the left placed loosely on the flat side of the pedal (the toe-clip was only on one side of the pedal) until I got moving.

Practising on the eight by ten concrete pad and lawn was awkward, so I attempted another street "launch." This time I sailed forward, but had a bit of trouble getting my foot in the toe-clip as it bounced around. Finally, I got it right. I followed a familiar route that was mostly flat, wide, paved trail. It was much safer than sharing the street with traffic and I confidently pedalled along. I noted with satisfaction my foot was no longer slipping. Biking was so much better than walking because I could enjoy the scenery and forget, for a short time, about my disability. I had given up busy roads, narrow mountain bike trails, and anything with steep hills because I did not trust my slower reaction time, but riding my safe, well-planned route gave me what I needed - fresh air, exercise, a sense of accomplishment, and the pure pleasure of being outdoors.

When I got home after twenty minutes of steady biking, however, my legs were so stiff they would barely move. I needed more resting and less accomplishing. I had to reprogram my thinking and remember it was not laziness but necessity. The same thing happened after shopping, doing errands, working, and even showering.

Rachel cut the lawn for me when she was home, but when I did it myself I managed by dividing the chore into smaller pieces. Cut the front lawn, then rest. Cut half the back lawn and rest. Cut the remainder and rest again. I often waited until late evening when it was cooler.

Amy moved out in July. She and Rachel trooped through the kitchen, loading out the last of her things. She handed me a gift bag.

"Here," she said shyly, "this is for you." Inside the bag was a thank-you card, and a stuffed "bear-angel" wrapped carefully in tissue paper.

"Thank-you, Amy. He's very sweet. I'm very proud of you for hanging in there to graduate. You'll never regret it." I gave her a big hug and Rachel waved as they walked out the door.

"See ya later, Mom." Rachel was ready to have her own space back. I was too.

~~~~~~

My brother Mike phoned.

"What are you guys doing towards the end of July? I want to make a road trip on my new bike and thought I might visit you." Mike had just acquired a Harley.

"We'll be around, and yeah, it would be great to see you. What route do you think you'll take?" It was about 1,000 km from Vancouver, through several mountain ranges.

"I'm not sure yet, but I'll probably take two days to get there. I've got a week off, and the kids will be in Osoyoos, so maybe I'll tie that in to my route plan on the way home."

It was so much fun going for rides on the back of the shiny motorcycle. The girls loved it, and I saw the area we lived in with new eyes. Rugged, wild, beautiful resource- filled land, rich with timber, oil and gas, and hard working, independent people.

All summer, I was careful to balance activity with rest, get lots of sleep, eat healthy food with plenty of fresh fruit and vegetables, and rebuild my tired immune system. When work began, I switched to afternoons hoping the later start would make a difference, but within a few days, it was a grind. I had trouble concentrating on helping the students.

From the minute I woke up in the morning until I went to bed, all my focus was on conserving energy. I dreaded the long hallways at school. I stopped carrying a water bottle around with me to drink so I would not have to walk the distance to the bathroom as much. The staffroom, where people I worked with shared stories, laughter, coffee and goodies, became too much effort to walk to in the short fifteen minutes we had at recess, so I took that time to sit in the classroom by myself and rest. People who were aware of how much I was struggling offered to run errands for me, and teachers who sometimes had aides to go and collect their class from the gym or music room were forced to do it themselves.

How many exceptions could be made? I already worked part-time, had no lunch or recess supervision, and now could not even perform simple tasks like using the photocopier or grabbing supplies from the work-room because of the distance. Carrying things with a cane was awkward and I was starting to feel as though I was not doing my job. What if I fell down the stairs or hurt a student? Just being on my feet for more than a few minutes at a time was stressful, and work became a gruelling marathon. My goal of working a few more years, at least did not factor in the extent or the rapid onset of fatigue. I knew it was not my fault. The disease was causing these problems, but I still felt like a failure. The biggest problem was that work was taking all my energy and I had nothing left to give to my family and my health problems. I was miserable.

At the end of November, my neurologist recommended I stop working altogether. The fight had gone out of me. I was frightened of the implications and prayed for mental as well as physical strength. Where was God now when I needed him? When would it stop? Was I headed for a wheelchair? Friends prayed for me.

Becky accepted my decision without many questions. She was slowly becoming more independent of me naturally, and this would simply speed the process along. I would be able to do a better job of caring for her with more rest and reduced stress. Rachel was perhaps a bit surprised, but she was compassionate, helpful and mature in her outlook. She knew I was still capable of a lot, and it did not occur to her to change her plans to move out of Hinton when she turned eighteen.

No matter what I did, said, or discussed with others, I was plagued with guilt. How could the woman who limped around using a cane still ride her bike or go swimming? If I could do those things, why couldn't I work? My thinking went in circles, defeating me before I had a chance to adjust to my new reality..

My close friend Bernadette lived in Calgary, where we had visited and stayed a few times, and we liked the big, modern city. I had always thought if I moved back to a city, it would be Vancouver, where we had friends, relatives and sense of belonging; but Vancouver was so far away, huge and expensive. It felt out of reach. Calgary was closer, had a reputable MS clinic, and we had good friends who lived there. Maybe change was the solution.

Kelly-Leigh came out west for her annual ski holiday, and treated the girls and me to a chalet at Jasper Park Lodge in the beautiful Rocky Mountains. French doors opened westward to a paved walking trail that followed beside a lake to the main lodge. After the skiers had departed for a day on the slopes, I started a fire in the fireplace and soaked in the warmth, fragrance and atmosphere of comfort in the wilderness. I stared at the flames and closed my eyes.

~~~~~~

I strained to raise my end of the canoe onto the roof rack, unconsciously scrunching my toes in an effort to pour more strength into my body.

"Come on, Kathy! It's just a canoe. Here, grab this cord, and we'll tie it down." Dave's impatience made my confusion even stronger, and later he pointed out my weakness again.

"Dan's wife lifted the canoe up there effortlessly. You need to get in better shape."

"She's a lot taller than me," I said defensively.

At that time, I blamed my lack of strength on stress and tiredness. We worked hard. So many insignificant memories had new meaning now.

~~~~~~

Rachel had a burning desire to "get out of Hinton." I was sad to see her go but I also recognized she needed to spread her wings, see the world from a new perspective, and make her own choices and mistakes. She chose to move to Red Deer with a girlfriend and in the early spring, the girls made the five-hour drive with the high hopes of youth and a fresh beginning in mind.

Change was in the air at our house and I jumped on board, wanting a clean start for my new, unexpected situation of stay-at-home mom. We targeted Calgary as our destination. Becky was keen on the idea of city life so I decided to take the risk. I listed our house for sale and made arrangements physically and mentally to move, but the house did not sell. Buyer after buyer looked at it, said they liked it, but did not make an offer.

It was a difficult summer. Every time we had an Open House it poured rain. Beforehand, I ran around making the house and yard look perfect to increase the odds of a sale. There were frequent showings, at awkward times, to add to the stress, and it was difficult to keep a routine with the interruptions. It helped when it was just the cats and I, but keeping them out of the way was a challenge. Sometimes they stayed out all night so I did not think anything of it when Bubbles was not around one morning. She would show up when she was hungry enough. My neighbour across the street came to the door before noon that day and asked if she could come in for a minute. We sat down at the table.

"Kathy, I have some bad news for you. Ray and I were standing in the garage this morning and noticed something lying on the road at the end of the driveway. We discovered it was your cat, Bubbles. She must have been hit by a car and killed. You know how fast the vehicles drive by here sometimes. I'm so sorry." She covered my hand with hers. Tears spilled down my face.

"Oh, Agnes, she was a beautiful cat, one of the nicest we've ever had. Becky's going to be devastated." Bubbles often visited our neighbours across the street.

"I know. We really enjoyed her too. She was very friendly. We wrapped her in a pink sheet and put her in our garage where it's cool while you decide what you want to do."

Agnes left, and I wandered around in a daze, thinking about keeping the cat until Becky arrived home from Ontario in a few days. I went outside to the shed and looked at the gardening shovel leaning against the wall. It was very hot. I needed to bury her right away, I soon realized. I called Agnes, and her husband brought the cat over in a cardboard box, with the pink sheet poking out. I was sitting on the back step when he arrived, and he put the box down beside me, pulled out his hanky, and dabbed at his nose. Ray was almost eighty. The care my neighbours showed and the sadness I felt washed down my face in a new flood of tears. After Ray left, I opened the box, looked in at the crushed body of our sweet cat and cried even more.

Early that evening I buried Bubbles in the nearby mountains. It was rocky ground but I dug a shallow grave and covered the box with dirt and a few wild flowers. God had given and God had taken away. My heart was heavy.

Family and friends knew we were moving. Becky thought she would not be returning to the same school in the fall so she said goodbye to friends. The housing market was booming in Hinton and many people sold and moved away quickly - I expected we would be one of those families. Time passed, and to prompt a sale, we dropped the selling price, twice. Towards the end of August an offer finally came in and with huge relief, I thought we would at last move forward, but the offer fell through.

A home inspection revealed insulation in the attic that posed a potential health risk, and the buyer withdrew his offer. The insulation was vermiculite, often used in older homes and it sometimes contained asbestos, I was told. There were other problems. The electrical wiring did not meet the current building codes, the roof was structurally questionable, and there were venting issues with the crawl space beneath the floor. I was flabbergasted. After eight years in the house, and a large chunk of money poured into upgrades and maintenance, how could all these problems have been missed?

~~~~~~

Rachel was facing her own set of challenges. After barely settling into Red Deer, she travelled to Europe for a two-month escapade, leaving her roommate behind to fend for herself.

"Mom, I need to come home. I thought I might stay in Europe longer, but I'm tired of being on my own, and I really miss my friends. I've seen what I wanted to see. The guy I'm working for here in Rome yells all the time and isn't happy with what I do. A whole bunch of us share a room, including him, and people are always coming and going. I want to quit. Even with working, I'll be out of money soon." After several frantic phone calls, I helped her change the flight date home by paying a small fee but things worsened. She phoned again.

"Oh Mom, Kim got evicted while I've been away, and I don't even have a place to come home to. On top of that she went to Calgary and I don't know what happened to my stuff." She started to cry.

"Wow. I'll try to find out where it is. In the meantime,

who's picking you up at the Calgary airport? Will you be working at Tim Horton's again?"

"Yes, I have a job. I think I have a ride from the airport to Red Deer but, Mom, where will I stay? This is such a nightmare. I'm so mad at Kim."

"Maybe someone at work could give you a couch to sleep on until you get things figured out. At least you have a job." I could feel my stress building. My own circumstances were causing me enough worry and confusion.

The next time Rachel phoned, it was from the Calgary airport.

"Mom, you'll never guess what happened. My friend got the dates mixed up. There's no one to pick me up and I'm stuck here! I just want to go home, but I don't even have a home to go to." Her voice broke. I wanted to jump in the car and help her through the mess, but it was too far away, too impractical, and we had other pressing commitments.

"Rachel, make some phone calls. Someone that you know might be able to help you out. Hang in there. Love you, bye." She made it to Red Deer that evening with the help of her smart, caring employers, and with persistence, Rachel found a place to live.

Asbestos - tiny airborne particles that if breathed in, could cause all kinds of health problems, invisible to the naked eye and potentially deadly. It could be in our home. The implications were staggering.

There was no one to deal with it locally, so I hired a remediation expert from Edmonton to take random samples of vermiculite from our attic for testing. Fine, silvery-gold particles the size of squished peas were carefully placed in labelled zip-lock bags by a man covered from head to foot in a white disposable suit,

234

masked and gloved. By then I knew that it would cost thousands of dollars to have the vermiculite removed from the attic if it was contaminated. Had our health been affected by this material? All week I waited for test results, praying the vermiculite would be asbestos-free, but steeling myself for the worst. The word I needed to hear echoed in my ear across the phone line. Negative. The vermiculite tested negative. The asbestos levels did not pose any health risks. I was freed of that huge worry.

An electrician came in and updated the wiring. The furnace and dryer were vented properly and the problems were slowly solved, cutting into my financial resources. I was tired of keeping the house and yard spotless but time was running out before winter began and Becky got settled into grade six. It seemed that when one problem was cleared up, another began. I needed to renew the real estate contract at the beginning of September. Was it worth continuing? Yes, I was not giving up that easily.

Warm, summer weather turned cool, and storm after storm brought heavy rains to the area. I walked by Becky's old bedroom and heard an unusual noise. It sounded like water dripping.

"Oh no, this can't be happening." Sure enough, a faint brown stain followed two white ceiling tiles to the corner where water pooled and a small drip had formed. I ran for a bucket. Within a few hours, I had three buckets out, in the bedroom, kitchen and mudroom. I phoned the real estate agent.

"I need to cancel the contract. The roof is leaking, and I cannot show the house like this. The venting isn't quite finished for the dryer, and who knows what else might be wrong." It was just too much. We were not meant to move right now. Relief poured through me and I relaxed for the first time in months.

A bit of roof caulking held the problem in check until the roof was re-shingled at the end of October, and I tried my hardest to be grateful for the blessings in my life over the Thanksgiving weekend. I had accepted the change in plans, trusting that God knew what we needed, even though I had not understood.

~~~~~~

At 3.30 pm on Tuesday afternoon following Thanksgiving, Mike called from Vancouver.

"Hey, Mike, how's it going?"

"Well, I've had better afternoons than this one." I heard him take a deep breath. "Paul was found dead in his apartment this morning." I fell onto the chair and gripped the phone hard. "Kathy, are you still there?"

"Yeah, I'm here. What happened to our brother?" My eyes remained dry and the tears would not come.

"Well, we won't know until some tests are done, but so far there's nothing obvious. Maybe it was his heart, maybe it was drugs, maybe it was booze." Open-heart surgery a few years before had fixed Paul up with a new valve, but there were no surgeries for drugs or alcohol.

"I talked to him last week, let's see, Wednesday night he phoned me. He was kind of pissed off, something about his phone being disconnected and we could reach him on his cell."

"Well, we invited him for a meal, since it was Thanksgiving and all, but we couldn't get hold of him. Guess that's why, if his phone was out."

"Were you there, at his apartment? Who found him?"

"Yeah, his friend Terry and his wife went over. They thought something was wrong because he didn't show up for work today. I went too, when they called. The place is a mess, really bad, Kathy. He'd stopped taking care of himself."

"He always hated cleaning, and I got the impression he was depressed lately."

"This was more than depressed. I really don't know what was going on; except it was evident he was drinking heavily the past while. There were bottles everywhere."

"Wow, I can't believe it. I'll get down as soon as I can." I hung up and sat motionless at the table. My brother was dead at forty-four years of age. It was unreal. My eyes stung and I wiped away the tears with a shaking, angry hand.

Another life taken by the bottle, sucked down into the pit of no return. The sad reality hit me hard. Even though the evidence pointed all along to alcohol, I wanted to believe otherwise, but there was no denying the disease had run its course and Paul had suffered an addiction he was powerless to control. Family history was repeating itself.

I was glad we did not know until after the funeral what had really taken my brother. It added a tiny bit of honour to the celebration of Paul's life. He would have liked the elegant chapel, the heartfelt speeches, the delicious food afterwards, but maybe not the minister's Biblical references and the overtly Christian theme. Paul was not a believer. The minister we met with beforehand was aware of this but we honoured our brother, nonetheless, filling the chapel with words and pictures that told the real story of Paul's life and brought laughter, smiles and tears to those who loved him and who had been touched by his life.

At the beginning of December, a large sum of money was deposited into my bank account, and I immediately phoned Mike.

"Did the life insurance money come through already? Wow, that's amazing." Paul was divorced, had no children and had named Mike as his beneficiary in the event of his death. Mike split this with me. It was another unreal event. I was forever grateful, to Mike, to Paul, and ultimately to God for changing the course of my future.

All of a sudden, the financial obstacle that stood in my way of moving back to the West Coast had been removed. Instead of Calgary, maybe I could consider Vancouver as an option.

~~~~~~

Dave unexpectedly moved to the west coast in the late fall. Becky had been spending time with her father on a regular basis for ten years, but he was suddenly going to be a thousand kilometres away instead of fifty. It was a big adjustment for both of them. It was ironic, really, that we had tried to move out of the area but Dave moved first, following his original goal only much delayed. I was happy for him.

My attention shifted to the housing market on the west coast and I searched for affordable housing for us on the outskirts of Vancouver, remembering my last impression of a place that had become very big, fast paced and unappealing to a "once-upon-a-time" city-girl. I was no longer that girl and remained uncertain of what was right for us.

Bernadette and I talked on the phone, excited about the Christmas season.

"We're going to be in Edmonton over the holidays, staying at a friend's place while they travel. They have a big house and Cathy said it would be fine if we had guests, so you and Becky would be welcome to come hang out with us for a couple of days."

"Rachel's coming up from Red Deer, but I think she has to go home on Boxing Day. Maybe we'll come then. It would be fun to do city stuff." I could hardly wait to see Rachel. We surprised her with a Christmas gift, a second-hand car. Our time together went swiftly.

Roads were free of snow on the highway drive to Edmonton. We planned a day with our friends at West Edmonton Mall Water Park, a huge indoor affair of pools, slides, lounging chairs and tons of glass that utilized the solar power of the bright, winter sun. The ceiling was many storeys above, built high to accommodate the variety of slides that had level after level of stairs and platforms. Green plants were spread throughout the big, airy space, making it much like an outdoor water park. It was amazingly warm. Groups of people gathered around the edge of the wave pool and concessions opened for business.

Our kids had boundless energy for the exciting slides. The day passed in a whirlwind of activity with smiles, screams and groans from some participants. The wave pool was as far as I got and I took Becky's hand for the first onslaught of waves. She soon disappeared with the boys for another round of slides and I stumbled through the water towards my recliner, willing myself more balance in the moving waves, eventually making it to the safety of the chair. We stayed until early evening. I followed Bernadette into the girls' change room carefully, using my cane as a security measure on the slippery, wet floor.

"Here's your stuff, Becky." Becky changed quickly and hurried out to meet the boys.

"I'm starving," Bern said as she pulled off her wet suit. "Let's stop for something to eat on the way home."

"Yes, let's do that. The kids are probably starving too. I wonder if..." I turned to walk down the narrow aisle and slipped in a pool of cold water. My cane flew out of my hand and I went down hard on the wooden bench. "Oooohhhhh, owwwwh." My left side caught the fall and I slid onto the bench as pain shot through me.

"Oh, Kathy, are you okay?" Bernadette's concerned face hovered nearby. I put a hand to my ribs while trying to straighten my spine.

"I really hurt my ribs but I'm okay." I winced in pain as I moved. Bernadette's eyes filled with tears and they spilled down onto her shirt.

"This stupid disease! I hate seeing you in pain. You're so brave."

"I hate it too. I hate limping around like a fool, not being able to do what most people can. Most of all I hate being tired all the time." My eyes watered as my friend leaned over and gingerly gave me a hug.

She waited for me to dress and gather my things, and stuck out her arm. I took it without speaking because I needed it. I was moved beyond words at Bernadette's compassion.

The pain made my eyes water. My jaw clenched. Andy drove my vehicle and I was grateful that my hunger pains dulled the ache in my ribs. The food tasted wonderful and we all ate like fiends. When we got back to the house, I took a painkiller and sat stiffly with a blanket, drifting into a restless sleep. Had I broken a rib?

The doctor suggested an x-ray would not change the management or the outcome of a rib fracture, which she thought I might have, and recommended rest and no lifting while the area healed.

I was slower than ever, but still upright. Not wanting to risk another fall in the icy winter conditions, I stayed home until the pain and bruising subsided. My frustration with my limited mobility mounted. At the end of the month, I was scheduled to see my neurologist.

"An orthotic would add stability to your walk. I recommend an appointment to see a specialist for this at the Glenrose Rehabilitation Hospital in Edmonton." I had gone to the well-known hospital in 1997 with Steven and his mother to see a host of specialists – doctors, a physiotherapist, and an occupational therapist who outlined what was best for Steven. Now it was my turn.

"All right, I guess I'm ready. I envisioned something heavy, bulky and uncomfortable, but what you've described sounds much better." I had held off on an orthotic for a few years, just like the cane, resisting the help, denying the need.

"From what you've described, it sounds as though the disease may have slipped into the next stage, what's referred to as secondary progressive. You've had no clinical relapses in over a year. So we'll monitor this and keep you on the interferon for now." I was frightened by what I had heard, but kept focusing on the fact that it was only "gradually worsening over time."

THIRTEEN

"In the Universe, there are things that
are known, and things that are unknown,
and in between, there are doors."
~ William Blake ~

One cold, snowy Saturday I flipped through a newspaper and stopped at the travel section.

"Hey, Becky, how would you like to go on a holiday somewhere soon? It's been years since I've been to Mexico. I bet Rachel would like to go, too."

"I'd like the vacation, I just don't know if I want to miss school." Unlike her older sister, Becky liked school very much.

The thought of a warm beach, someone else cooking, a relaxed pace after the stresses of the past eight months, plus the financial resources to do this, tempted me to look closely each Saturday at vacation packages. Rachel had just settled into a work routine after extra time off to fly to Vancouver for Paul's funeral and had trouble booking a full week off. Becky had school until spring break in March.

I was beginning to push the idea aside when an ad for a vacation package to Victoria BC got me thinking about the coast again. I had travelled to Vancouver Island years before and spent a summer working on a forestry research project that kept us moving around on the south half of the Island, which was beautiful. It would not be beach weather in March, but at least we would have a break from snow and cold temperatures, and we could see if we liked Victoria. I booked two tickets.

The plane descended and suddenly I could see water. The left wing dipped towards the ocean as we turned southward. Rounded forested mountains with rocky outcrops reminded me this was coastal landscape, bursting with vegetation, cedars and firs dripping moss like an old man's beard, and the odd snow-covered peak. The snow was a surprise, but to my relief it stayed in the mountains where, as my Dad used to say, it should. Vancouver was the only place in the world where you could boat, golf and ski all in the same day. His words echoed in my mind. We walked down the stairs from the plane onto the tarmac, unhindered by the icy cold of Alberta and I breathed in the moist ocean air. I could not wait to see more.

We stayed downtown in the Inner Harbour, half a block from the stately Parliament Buildings, with ocean vistas, museums, restaurants and shops surrounding us. Spring blossoms were everywhere, fountains were spilling water, and horse-drawn carriages sat waiting quietly for their next excursion about town. Boats of all sizes sat serenely on the water, gulls squawked, horns sounded, and people went about their business in the midst of orderly clamour. We spent two days exploring the fairy-tale setting, and two days with a real estate agent touring different areas and looking at a few condos for sale. Housing was pricey.

"Do you think we'll move to Victoria, Mom?" Becky asked on the trip home.

"I'd like to, Becky. Would you like that?"

"Um, I think so. When would we move?"

"Ideally, in the summer, but I haven't got that far in

my planning. We have to sell the house first, and you know what happened last summer. So, we'll see." I was dreading listing the house again even though the market was still strong.

I toyed with the idea of selling our house without a realtor, and went as far as talking to my lawyer and picking up a few copies of a purchase contract. I wanted to be prepared for different options despite my doubts. My neighbour had actually stopped in and asked if I still wanted to sell the house, so that was encouraging. It at least prompted me to get started.

On a rainy weekend in early May, before I had made any decisions to list the house with a real estate company, two offers to purchase arrived within twenty-four hours. Two offers! I had only picked up the contracts the day before and bumbled my way through filling them out, not wanting to jeopardize a sale. When I phoned my neighbour with the news that there had been an unexpected offer from a teacher I knew, she and her husband made a slightly higher offer, even though I had already accepted the first one. It was beyond my understanding. I was ecstatic.

The waiting began. As on most property sales, there were a few conditions to be met before the sale was finalised. The buyers were concerned about sewage backup problems, and paid to have the pipes tested. I sweated a bit, given the unexpected problems from the year before, but the lines were clean and the results reflected that. I provided the buyers with copies of all the recent work done, including a re-shingled roof and a clean bill of health from the insulation examination. Victoria was beginning to look like a real possibility when the deal fell through at the last minute. The buyers could not get financing.

All was not lost, however, because there was a backup offer. Two weeks of waiting turned into four, but this time all was well and the sale proceeded smoothly. On confirmation of "sold," I sprang into action. Victoria was now the focus and I booked flights to the capital city. We needed a place to live. Rachel had been following the events closely from Red Deer.

"Mom, do you think I could come with you guys? I might consider moving if things don't work out here." I was thrilled with her interest.

"Of course, if you can get a few days off. We'll be gone about four days. We could meet in Edmonton."

"Okay, I'll call you back as soon as I find out. Did I tell you I have a new boyfriend?"

"No, you didn't. What's his name?"

"Logan. I'll tell you more later, but I have to go, so I'll talk to you soon. Bye."

We flew out of the Edmonton airport and landed in Calgary to change planes. I groaned when I saw the distance we had to walk in the big, busy airport.

"My legs will be done in by the time we get to Victoria. Gosh, this is frustrating."

"Just wait here, Mom. I'll be right back." I watched Rachel disappear the way we had come and remembered the time she just had to have a burger before we continued travelling. We had lots of time. Becky followed her sister and I sat down on a bench to rest. My legs were shaky. It had been a busy, exciting month with lots more to come. I was just beginning to wonder what the girls were up to when I spotted Rachel pushing an empty wheelchair towards me.

"Get in, Mom. It'll save your strength for Victoria." This was a first for me, but I was not about to argue. I had a very astute daughter.

It was a long way, and when we got to a carpeted, slow descending ramp way, Rachel yelled, "Hold on" and pushed as fast as she could. The excitement bug bit me as I forgot about my frustration with limited mobility. We stopped at an open area restaurant for a meal and I struggled to get out the wheelchair. Rachel put her hand on my shoulder.

"Why don't you stay put, Mom? Look, I can push you right up to a table. I'll go and get us something to eat while you and Becky wait here." I relaxed. It was okay to be dependant on others. I remained in the chair until we boarded the plane, where we got special treatment, boarding before everyone else. Maybe this was not so bad after all!

We were whisked around the city with the help of a realtor. Limited choice in our price range quickly narrowed the process and I made an offer twenty-four hours before flying home. It was a new lifestyle choice for us - a third-floor condo with a wide-open floor plan, laminate floors, and a balcony, surrounded with lots of trees and flowers. The small building had an elevator, short walking distances, and privacy.

There were so many things I was unsure about, details I did not think of until after we got home. It all seemed so perfect when we were there. There was no grass to cut, driveway to shovel, rugs or stairs to trip over. I worried about the neighbourhood, the busy street, traffic, noise and the people. I was not even certain that disability funding from my employer would follow me out of the province. It was a time for risks and a time to trust God. Within a week, the sale had gone through. I began the details of planning a move, collecting boxes, making phone calls and finding a mover. It was all happening very fast. In the midst of all the excitement, I almost forgot an important appointment in Edmonton for an AFO, the ankle-foot orthotic I had long resisted. I kept thinking of it as a UFO, which kept me chuckling to myself for the entire drive to the hospital.

The specialist introduced herself.

"How do you spell physiatrist?" This was a specialist in physical and rehabilitation medicine. There were so many different specialists, I was losing track.

"All the information you need will be in the letter I'll send to your neurologist. Let's go over what I know so far." Soon I was walking the length of the hallway outside the exam room as she observed my gait, turning and moving with and without the cane. She did more tests of strength and reflexes on the examining table. We discussed exercise, stiffness and management of spasticity. I told her of our recent decision to move to Victoria as she wrote out a prescription.

"I don't think an orthotic can be made before you move, so I'll forward some names and phone numbers of places in Victoria that can make it for you."

"Thank you. I'll make an appointment as soon as we get settled."

Rachel called me the following afternoon. We had parted at the Edmonton airport the week before when she returned to Red Deer. I wondered if she would move with us to Victoria.

"Hi Mom. You'll never guess what happened. It was scary. My car caught on fire and burned up. I lost my purse, CDs and some clothes. It was really scary."

"What! Are you okay?"

"I'm fine, and Logan's fine. We're just shaken up about it. The fire department came, and lots of people crowded around and watched. It caused a huge commotion." Thank goodness she wasn't by herself.

"What happened?" I bought that car for her. We had had it inspected at a local repair shop and everything was fine at the time but there were no guarantees with second hand cars, and this one was ten years old with an uncertain history.

"We were driving on the highway and there was this rattling from the front end. I thought something was wrong, so we pulled off outside the town of Stettler on a service road and drove into the parking lot of Tim Horton's. There was smoke coming from somewhere in the front of the car, and we stopped and jumped out to take a look. The tire blew off and we could see flames. A man came running over and told us to get away in case the car exploded, and to leave our stuff in the car. By the time the fire department got there, the car was badly burned." She took a deep breath.

"So where's the car?"

"It got towed away. It's damaged beyond repair. We were stuck there until a friend came to pick us up. Mom, do you think you could phone and ask about insurance, since we set it up in Hinton?"

"Sure, I'll phone right away and let you know what I find out. I'm just glad you're okay." I hung up and wondered about my daughter's bad luck with vehicles. This was the second in a year and a half. Maybe she was not meant to have her own.

Goodbyes are always hard. It was an action-packed, emotional month for Becky and me. Even Rachel, who had moved to Red Deer, said she no longer felt as though she had a home to go to, but that did not stop us from moving on. I knew it was time to go. A door had been opened, wide. Rachel could always join us if it did not work out in Red Deer. We would make room.

We had plenty of help. At the beginning, I felt organized but as the month progressed, I was overwhelmed by all the details, and had forgotten how exhausting a big move was. We drove out of Hinton with a truckload of stuff, Victoria bound.

Our stressed out cat did not understand what was

going on and when we reached Kamloops for our first stopover, Missy hid under the bed in the hotel room. It was very hot and we kept the vehicle air-conditioning on full blast. Without it, I would not have been able to function. My legs did not want to work in the oppressive heat and Becky often stuck out her arm to support me. She had seen my good friends Kelly-Leigh and Bernadette do the same.

Settling into Victoria took some time. Everything was new and I had just spent the last 23 years of my life in West Central Alberta in the "boonies." Becky had never lived anywhere else. Even the cat was freaked out. She jumped off the third floor balcony when we first arrived and I thought for sure we had lost yet another cat but she showed up at the front door of the building twenty-four hours later, happy to find us and make a new home.

There were more stresses to deal with - our furniture and personal belongings did not arrive for three weeks, and the condo had some maintenance issues with plugged drains and ill-fitting water pipes. We were blessed with great neighbours and tried to live one day at a time. Becky and I took advantage of the empty space and painted her bedroom lime-green. My parents used to use the word *hideous* when they really did not like something, but I kept my mouth shut. We explored the city and went to the beach and several beautiful parks. The weather was gorgeous and continued so well into fall.

Becky started grade seven at a nearby school a few minutes' walk away. She was nervous at first but made friends quickly. My time was occupied with detail after detail and I tried to keep pace with all the changes, grateful for the move, a mild climate, a functioning home, and a new community to explore.

"Let's go to the pool, Becky. I hear the water's amazingly warm and there are some fun sprinklers to splash around in." I quashed my fear of slipping on the pool deck by wearing water shoes and was impressed by the locker room that was set up to accommodate wheelchairs. It was user friendly from my perspective. Becky laughed in the figure-eight shaped "play pool" as water jets pushed her around. The water was indeed warm. I hoped to start swimming lengths again at some point.

We had found a new church "home" that was welcoming and I hoped Becky would make some new friends through their youth group. At school, she was the "new kid" but did not seem to mind and brought home the usual stack of newsletters and forms for parents. We were invited to a family barbeque to meet some of the teachers.

"You don't have to come, Mom. I know all our teachers already."

"But it's for the parents too, Becky. I'd like to go."

"Aw, Mom do you have to? Just forget about it." I was puzzled by her reaction, but determined to go. I discovered she did not want to be seen with me.

"Mom, I don't want my friends to see your cane."

"Oh, I see. It didn't matter in Hinton."

"Yes, but they knew you and got used to it. It makes you look old, like a Grandma."

I was silent. I needed time to think about this. Was Becky ashamed of me?

I marked the date of the barbeque on the calendar and thought maybe I could try going without my cane for a day and see what it was like. We had sliding mirror doors in the hallway and when Becky was at school, I practised walking "freestyle." I forced myself to go shopping and run errands without the cane and discovered it was a scary world on my own two shaky legs. I had had some nasty falls. Somehow, along the way the cane had become a friend, something to help me along the way. It was part of me and I could not just leave it behind because Becky did not like the image it portrayed.

The school morning was sunny and warm. As Becky got ready for class, I sat at the kitchen table with a cup of coffee.

"What time is the barbeque, Becky?"

"I'm not sure. You don't need to come, you know. Lots of my friends are going by themselves."

"Well, I'd like to meet some of your teachers, so I'm going. Here, the notice says five o'clock. I guess I'll see you after school." The door slammed as Becky left. I was sad. When had image become such a big deal?

I shuffled around the apartment and as the morning progressed, so did my exhaustion. My legs felt peculiar, like a tiny puncture in a tire with air slowly leaking out, eventually causing the tire to collapse. Usually, when I sat a lot it helped build up some strength, but this time when I stood up at lunchtime, there was nothing left in my legs and I collapsed back onto the chair. This had never happened before without over-exertion.

I crawled down the hallway to my bedroom where the computer chair was tucked up to the desk and with the strength of my arms, pulled myself into the seat and swivelled around. I could still move my legs, and pushed the chair-on-wheels out into the hall with my feet. Once I was on the laminate floor it was easy to move about.

When Becky arrived home at three o'clock, I was still in the chair. She did not notice anything unusual, so I continued to work at the computer until hunger drove me to the kitchen.

"What are you doing, Mom? Why are you using the computer chair in the kitchen?"

"Well, Beck, my legs have decided to quit working today so you get your wish. I won't be going to the barbeque."

"Oh. Well, I guess I'll walk up to the school soon and meet my friends."

"That would be fine. The computer chair has come in handy today. I sure hope the strength to walk comes back into my legs."

"Uh-huh. What time is it?" The phone rang and Becky disappeared into her room.

She left shortly after. I pushed the chair around in the kitchen using the microwave to heat a pasta dinner and retreated to the couch to watch the news. By bedtime, I could tell my legs were recovering from the mysterious shutdown, but I stayed off my feet anyway as a precaution. The following day was business as usual and I stood up after a restful sleep with confidence and strength.

The ankle-foot orthotic was made in the late fall after I had gone for a couple of fittings. When the technician made the mould, he had covered the bottom of my foot from my toes up to the groove behind my left knee. Once made, the thin, light plastic that cupped my foot, heel and calf was held in place by a strong Velcro strap at the ankle and just below the knee. It was surprisingly comfortable, and by taking the insole out of my left shoe, the orthotic slid into the shoe easily and there was enough room for my foot. He recommended a larger shoe size but I resisted the idea and insisted on squishing my size-seven foot, with the orthotic, into a size-seven shoe. At first, it was a minor discomfort, as the brace provided me with stability, confidence and less tendency to trip. Over time, I switched to a size eight shoe when I discovered the left foot was indeed cramped and sore after prolonged use. Becky would not be seen with me in public, even though it was hidden under my pants.

Swimming was my next challenge. I wore my water shoes to prevent slipping and observed a high proportion of users who were in the same category as me. They were stiff and awkward, using whatever aid they needed to move around. It had been over two years since I had swum any laps after a "frozen shoulder" that plagued me the previous winter, but it was time to try again. I didn't feel safe riding a bicycle on the busy city streets and no longer owned a bike. Swimming was safer and I enjoyed the warm water.

A dozen laps was a good start. I did not want to overdo it and not be able to walk afterwards, thinking about the swimming instructor's warning, "Don't quit for months and expect to pick up where you left off." With energy to spare, I carried on with my day, satisfied and relieved I could finally do something to get regular exercise that did not take all my energy and a big chunk of time. I continued once a week, adding two laps until I built up to twenty. In the past, swimming had taken a huge amount of effort, and required rest along every step of the way, and further rest at home. Now I did not have to wait at all. What a breakthrough!

It actually rained in October, after three months of steady sun and blue skies. We laid Paul's ashes to rest on Thanksgiving in the North Vancouver Cemetery with Dad's ashes, one year after his death. I tried not to think of it as a tragedy and once again, my sorrow poured out onto the page in a sad poem.

The following week, I met with a neurologist at the MS Clinic in Victoria, and we scheduled an MRI for the New Year. The words "secondary progressive" were mentioned again, and this time I paid more attention. I learned it did not necessarily mean things would get worse. It simply meant the course of the disease had changed and could do anything at that point - improve, worsen, stay the same but not disappear altogether. This was news to me. I thought progressive meant a downhill ride, but trusted the doctor's opinion that this was not always the case. In the meantime, he recommended continuing the drug I was on, which I had already resigned myself to using indefinitely.

A freak snowstorm hit the west coast at the beginning of December that sent the city into a tailspin of closures, accidents, power outages and panic. The brunt of the storm was felt in Vancouver where hectares of Stanley Park were destroyed by high winds. Huge old trees toppled in the exposed landscape and the famous seawall where I had walked years before sustained massive damage. A large portion of the park remained closed for months afterwards. We had our share of fallen trees, icy roads and downed wires on the Island, and after four days at home, I ventured out into the parking lot to find the car doors iced shut. It took almost an hour to get onto the road. The cold, wintery weather lasted ten days. The storm broke records and locals said they had not experienced anything like it for years. I was used to harsh winters, but was surprised to experience them on the coast.

During the winter months, I continued to explore the city, getting lost, making new discoveries and enjoying every moment behind the wheel of my sporty little Mazda. The antiquated SUV had no role in my new city lifestyle and I had happily traded it in. The privilege of driving had been mine for most of my life and kept the world wide open, accessible and convenient, something many of us take for granted, like walking.

We slowly rebuilt an inventory of healthcare professionals and I made optometry appointments for both Becky and myself. So far, my eyes had remained unaffected by a chronic illness that was known to play havoc with vision so I had no indication that anything could be wrong.

Unlike the dentist, I looked forward to eye exams because it often meant new glasses. For years, I had worn contacts and kept old glasses hidden in a drawer to wear in a pinch. I had recently switched to glasses, partly out of choice, but mostly because I could not see properly with my contacts. Distance was fine, but close up work was impossible. Once I got used to wearing glasses, it seemed like a lot less fuss than contacts and I started paying attention to the variety of styles people were wearing. I wanted to update my huge, old glasses that weighed a ton on my face and looked very old fashioned.

I subjected myself to the usual battery of tests and consented to have irritating eye drops put into my eyes, all in the name of perfect eye health, so when the technician hesitated and had me redo the peripheral vision test because I missed seeing some of the blinking dots on the screen, I sensed something amiss. The optometrist performed further tests before giving me her opinion.

"Is everything okay?" I asked. "I got the impression there might be something wrong." I held my breath. Vision had suddenly become critically important.

"There appears to be some inconsistencies in the left eye, particularly in your peripheral line of vision, so I'm going to refer you to a specialist for further testing."

"You mean there might be some damage from MS to my left eye?"

"It's a possibility." Her voice remained level.

"Could it affect my driving? Will I lose my licence?" Panic had entered my voice.

"It could. The province is very strict about vision requirements, but I really can't say for sure until you have more detailed tests."

I left the office with my eyes stinging from the dye, blinking in the bright sunlight, fear pouring through me. My mind was clouded with doubt, worry and anguish over the next four months as tests and appointments came and went. My life would change forever if I could not drive. I enjoyed driving and I depended on driving to get me where I needed to go. But what, God forbid, if I hit someone, had an accident, or hurt Becky or myself? Self-pity engulfed me in its tenacious grip.

Rachel helped me see a new perspective. My twenty-year old daughter had maturity beyond her years and she listened, coached, counselled and empathized with me.

"Mom, I've had some really bad experiences with vehicles. I'd rather take the bus, or let someone else drive. It wouldn't be that bad. You could get one of those electric scooters and still get out, year round, in the west coast climate. Besides, you don't even know for sure what the results will be."

"Worry: to be uneasy or anxious; to fret." The worry was often all for naught, but most of us are susceptible to that nagging little voice inside that can make life a misery. Fortunately, I was not usually a chronic worrier, but this problem got under my skin.

The specialist ushered me into his office. I had built up a wall of defence that tumbled down as I heard him speak.

"We've detected a small amount of damage to your left eye from multiple sclerosis. That being said, it's not enough to impede your day-to-day vision judgment."

"Everything you've told me sounds positive, but does this mean I can still drive without endangering myself or others?"

"Yes, you meet all the criteria. You may need to get a driver's medical periodically, but your doctor will decide that with you."

I wanted to shout, sing and dance with joy. The sun had come out again. I could still drive. I had won this fight, but the experience taught me to take nothing for granted. God had decided I needed to sweat a little before hearing the good news.

My legs continued to carry me through the days and I kept up swimming and stretching until the following June. I met the neurologist regarding the results from the MRI. "The disease appears inactive at the time of the test and from everything you've described in the past year. Until this point, I would say it has entered the secondary progressive stage."

"So *inactive* means damage has stopped? I might not get any worse?"

"Yes, sometimes it just burns out for unknown reasons. There are no guarantees for the future, but for now it's inactive." He hesitated. "So the medication you're taking is no longer doing anything because of this. Some patients are nervous about stopping the injections in fear that if they stop, things will worsen. They likely will not worsen. Take your time and think about it and perhaps in six months we can do another MRI to confirm the inactivity. At that point I would recommend you go off the interferon." My eyes widened in surprise.

"Can I just stop the injections? Now? No more needles?" He smiled kindly.

"That's right. If you want to ask the MS nurse more

about it on your way out, she has lots of experience with this and can give you excellent advice."

I stopped in at her office and spent the next half-hour discussing various concerns I had.

"You know, Kathy, some people even feel a little bit better after they quit the meds, with a little less stiffness and a bit more energy. You can call me anytime if something comes up you're wondering about." She was a warm, knowledgeable woman who listened to my worries and long list of complaints with genuine compassion.

"The hardest part for me in the past year has been my almost-teenage daughter's rejection of my slow ways. She frequently points out all my faults and doesn't want to be seen with me. She says I embarrass her." My status of "cool mom" had dropped to "loser" before my very eyes. We had frequent fights, and she had all but cut me out, preferring the company of her friends. The name-calling hurt the most - labels like lame, slow, forgetful and worst of all, old. I laughed away some of it, agreed with some of it and explained to Becky how mean and hurtful it was to anyone. The nurse nodded.

"It's a hard age, no matter what the circumstances. It happens to lots of parents. The trick is to not take it all personally, ignore some of it, and know that it will pass. I have a magazine for teens that have parents with MS she might identify with. I'll send that home with you."

"Thanks so much. It's really helped talking to you. It makes me realize I don't talk much about having MS with anyone."

"You can contact the MS Society, you know. They have some excellent programs, informal coffee drop-ins, and an exercise program." I stood up and shook her hand.

"Thanks again. Bye." I walked out the door with

lightness in my step I had not felt for years. I had already decided the medication was history. Why would I take a drug that was not doing any good?

The nurse was right. I did feel a bit better, emotionally as well as physically. It took another six months for me to notice that I actually gained energy as I swam and that my legs felt that adrenaline rush of life-giving force. My daughter nonchalantly offered the support of her arm in public one day, the name-calling subsided, and "old" was substituted by "pretty." My trips to the pool showed me that disability hit people of all ages much worse than me. It was humbling.

FOURTEEN

"Faith means … knowing that something is real
even if we do not see it."
~ Hebrews 11:15 ~

A folded aluminum lawn chair in my left hand, book
and water bottled tucked safely into the webbing, with
cane gripped firmly in my right hand, I carefully picked
my way around large, weathered driftwood through
soft sand. Unsteady on my legs, at the first level spot I
threw my cane down, popped open the chair and
plunked down. Now I could really take it all in. Waves
broke on the shore, gulls cried to each other, and
children's voices carried in the warm breeze.

My gaze drifted across a large expanse of ocean
southward to the Olympic Mountains, where tips were
brushed with snow as if randomly stroked with an
artist's paintbrush. I watched a large ship turn into a
tiny dot and disappear. Two slow-moving barges
traversed the water, a small powerboat slapped the
waves, and to the east, a colourful sailboat emerged
from the bay where a historic lighthouse stood among
the rocks. Two women walked by with a large dog that
bounded in and out of the water joyfully and I felt only
a tiny amount of envy at their seemingly effortless

energy. I had come with the intention of walking a stretch of the beach myself but I knew my legs needed rest rather than more activity, so I decided my eyes would do the walking for me today.

It was so beautiful here. To the west, the water sparkled and danced as the sun shone a path of light across the surface. I closed my eyes and soaked in the tranquillity.

Eventually, I opened my book but could not concentrate on the words. A man jogged beside the water, a dog his willing partner, and two young children dug in the sand, chattering to each other as a watchful mother sat on a towel nearby. It reminded me of days gone by with my own children. Feelings of nostalgia washed over me. I had been so fit, so strong, so capable, and now it was all gone, or was it? I was as fit as I could be given the circumstances. In what sense did I want to be strong? My physical capacity was diminished by disease, but I felt strong mentally. Spiritually, God gave me steady strength. The physical strength I did possess I put to good use most of the time. In what way was I not capable? Once again, my thoughts centered on the physical. My life was still rich, full and blessed, even though it was not what I expected it to be. My thoughts became philosophical as I stared at the giant kelp with their over-inflated onion-like blobs bouncing on the surface of the water.

Illness is not often a measured, tangible object. Visible, like the water in front of me, invisible like the life hidden below the surface, it constantly changes like the ocean, mixing things around and playing havoc with body, mind and spirit. It is a challenge to stay balanced in this turmoil of change but like the creatures in the ocean, we need to find our niche in order to continue.

Staying strong physically, mentally and spiritually is paramount to our well-being. For me, withdrawal into my own private world to regroup, rejuvenate, pray and write it down allows me to float to the surface and reach out to others.

I heard a bark, and my eyes travelled down the beach to where the jogger stopped to throw a stick into the water. His dog began an enthusiastic paddle to obtain his prize and soon dropped the stick at his master's feet, waiting with ears pricked for the next throw. That's it, I thought. We need to be ready and willing to give, receive and help in whatever way we can, no matter what our circumstances.

A friend once told me I was a survivor, but I prefer the label "fighter." Beneath the skin, hidden from view, is a boxing ring where cells duke it out day after day, slamming each other down until the buzzer sounds and victory or defeat is declared. Even on the down days, I pull myself up and stagger about for yet another round. I'm a sore loser. With today's medical advances, faith, family and a host of good friends cheering me on, the odds are in my favour for a winning round - I press onward for the prize...

ISBN 142518665-3

9 781425 186654